# THE DEFINITIVE SEX GUIDE FOR COUPLES

## 2 BOOKS IN 1

**SAMANTHA MAY**

The information provided herein is stated to be truthful and consistent, in that any liability, in terms of inattention or otherwise, by any usage or abuse of any policies, processes, or directions contained within is the solitary and utter responsibility of the recipient reader. Under no circumstances will any legal responsibility or blame be held against the publisher for any reparation, damages, or monetary loss due to the information herein, either directly or indirectly. Respective authors own all copyrights not held by the publisher.

The information herein is offered for informational purposes solely, and is universal as so. The presentation of the information is without a contract or any type of guarantee assurance. The trademarks that are used are without any consent, and the publication of the trademark is without permission or backing by the trademark owner. All trademarks and brands within this book are for clarifying purposes only and are owned by the owners themselves, not affiliated with this document.

# Table of Contents

# INTRODUCTION

Sex and women's sexuality are subjects that are fraught with emotion. Often women feel ashamed talking about the sexual needs of theirs and also search for all kinds of secret dishes to compensate for it. Nevertheless, sex is a proper activity that offers a heap of benefits! It can help keep the body of your own and mind as lively as you age. While the pastime is beneficial and healthy for both genders, you can find specific health bonuses that just benefit women.

The advantages of sex for women include:

Reduced blood pressure
Far better immune system
Good heart health, perhaps including reduced risk for heart disease
Enhanced self-esteem
Decreased anxiety and depression
Improved libido
Immediate, natural pain relief
Much better sleep
Increased closeness and intimacy to a sexual partner
General emotional stress reduction, both physiologically as well as Women that are emotional, obviously, have a number of various lifestyles, situations, and preferences with regards to sex. Thankfully, most women are able to feel the benefits of sex, regardless of the situation of theirs.

## BENEFITS OF SEX FOR WOMEN

## 1. Lowers Stress

Many women's health issues are a consequence of stress, with an example being heart problems. Thankfully, sex might be in a position to help and be an excellent stress-reliever. During sex, your brain 's pleasure centers are struck with dopamine while the cortisol level drops of your own. Oxytocin, which boosts feelings of friendship as well as happiness is released in droves. When you are stressed out, this particular chemical cocktail that rushes into your brain when you are having intercourse is just what you have to calm the mood of your own. And also you can never ever have sufficient endorphins, right?

## 2. Boosts your immune system

Pennsylvania's Wilkes Faculty research center discovered that college pupils who had sex at least one time a week had higher degrees of immunoglobulin A in the saliva of theirs. Immunoglobulin A is an antibody that can help your body deal with dangerous foreign invaders and go on following a proper lifestyle.

Sex can improve your body's serotonin level also. This particular hormone can help generate "happy feelings", and researchers think that there is a link between depression and also the body's serotonin amount.

## 3. Lowers your blood pressure

High blood pressure is able to have a really good impact on the health of your own. It is able to lead to serious or even fatal cardiovascular complications. Study shows that hypertension can in fact impact a women's potential to orgasm! And sex was connected to good aerobic consequences in women in addition to lower systolic blood pressure readings.

## 4. You rest better

A satisfying round of sex is able to enable you to battle insomnia. When your body reaches orgasm, it is started with a wave of prolactin, a hormone that encourages relaxation. And research suggests that sex triggers the generation of a lot more prolactin compared to masturbation does.

## 5. Increased libido

Higher libido is related to many benefits, for instance, it contributes to the self-esteem of your own as well as pain resistance. You will feel a lot more desire to have your partner which can turn into being much more desired yourself. You will find reasons why many people want to be hooked up to the sexual nature of theirs.

## 6. Improves cardio health

Sex and health are directly linked. Women who reported having a pleasurable sex life experienced a reduced risk of other problems and hypertension. The study's authors posit that having a lot of happy sex is great for the heart of your own. It might be because a women's sexual satisfaction with the partner of her is usually connected to her improved mental well-being.

## 7. Trains your pelvic floor

Pelvic floor muscles that are accountable for controlling the urine flow of your own may be weakened naturally through age or even by pregnancy. And in case you have previously peed while laughing, it is since you have to exercise them much more. During sex, these muscle groups are going to get an excellent exercise. You are able to exercise them by yourself, but what fun is the fact that when there are plenty of positions for two?

## 8. Creates intimacy

Maybe unsurprisingly, researchers have discovered that sex creates affection and intimacy in relationships. The greater number of sex some has, the more they feel connected to one another. Pro research suggests that actual physical affection and touch are really important, quite possibly for couples that happen to be together for many years.

## 9. Protects the brain of your own

Women who remained sexually active into older age had far better cognitive functioning compared to people who ceased fooling around. Researchers measured the women's potential to remember words and adjusted the end result to account for factors as depression and also the women's physical activity level. Sexually active women performed better on the test.

## 10. Skin burns calories

Both women and men burn fat during bedroom romps. You get to stretch out your move and body in uncommon ways. You will not burn up a load of calories, some estimates place it from five calories a minute, though you will remain energizing the body of your own

# THE BEST WAY TO ATTRACT MEN

**1. Manage The Mood of your own**
Making your mood a priority is likely to be an enormous win for you with regards to being more appealing
Why?
Men are instinctively attracted to women that are happy. When you're in a great mood, he can feel this satisfying vibe when he's around you.
Men are able to sense the vibe of your own and also you do not need to point out anything to really make it come across; in fact, the less you "try" to "prove" what a great mood you're in and also the more you concentrate on just being in a great mood, the more well off you'll be.

**2. Have Fun**
Do things you like. Take time out to do entertaining items in the life of your own in

which you are able to let loose and truly laugh and enjoy with things.

No matter whether it is heading away with buddies and also getting a very good time or maybe passing time with loved ones and living life in a happy, enjoyable way. Experience life in the second and do not obsess with little things that do not matter.

If you genuinely have fun and are happy, this automatically makes you more attractive to men. Men are drawn to women that are happy who could laugh a whole lot and therefore are happy. Do not fake it; this will come off as fake and will not be sexy.

## 3. Do Not Compare Yourself To Other Women

I comprehend the instinct to compare yourself to various other women and also to various other individuals on the whole. Perhaps you see second women and also you believe to yourself, "if just I'd ...." (insert whatever it's you want you can change about yourself that she has).

Take this particular mindset and set it aside.

The main reason I'm saying to you This is as whenever you compare yourself, almost all you should do is make yourself feel frustrated and miserable. The very best thing to perform is to be the best self of your own & concentrate on things you are able to control as well as improve upon. This can make you feel very good.

## 4. Do What Feels Comfortable

You may have read that using a wacky outfit, getting an unusual sex toy contraption or even doing a bit of very sensual as well as risque is the sole method to draw in men.

Overlook all of this particular. Trying to "do things" which you're totally uncomfortable with since you feel it is going to attract men is a terrible idea since you won't be at ease.

Being more comfortable is important with regard to being appealing to men. In case you're comfy, you are going to find that all you do is organically as well as effortlessly much more appealing to men.

And so do not think that you've to do anything that causes you to feel unnatural and awkward because it will not assist you anyway.

## 5. Know Yourself

Self-discovery is a continuing practice which all of us go through in the lives of ours. We're constantly growing and changing as individuals.

This is a crucial step with regards to being attractive: get to find out yourself almost as you are able to and this will instantly allow you to feel more self-confident and comfy.

What I mean by realizing yourself is to know your weaknesses and strengths and be in a position to identify what you're good at and everything you are not obviously good at.

These mindsets are going to automatically make you more attractive to men.

How The Appearance of your own Will Attract The Men You Want

Obviously physical appearance is a subject that needs to be addressed with regards to making men attracted to you.

It is a very fact of life: human beings and men are visual creatures. You will find specific things men will respond to whether he really wants to or not. I am just providing you with this info to help you... never to offend or even be rude, and so please

## 6. Makeup

Every man has various preferences with regards to makeup, but there's a regular theme with what most men appear to find sexy.

Me personally, I love it when a woman throws in an endeavour to complete makeup which enhances just how she currently looks but doesn't pile on the base after which add a lot of various powders as well as whatnot to it.

I've noticed women using all those massive fake eyelashes for instance after which a load of fake tanner on and too much makeup it was apparent from a mile away... and I suppose a few men do discover this particular hot but many would rather a small amount less.

With which said, an excellent program of makeup may change a women's look so certainly do not hesitate to apply makeup.

## 7. Fitness/Diet

This is a really sensitive subject and I do not want anybody to get offended and point out I'm attempting to point out all women need to be skinny.

This is false at all. Everything I'm saying is the fact that staying as healthy as you potentially can and making good diet options (good eating options not starving) is the primary key to looking your best.

Listen to the body of your own do not attempt to look the way you obviously cannot look without needing to starve or even be unhealthy. This is crucial. Good is sexy.

## 8. Clothing

Clothing is able to make a huge difference with regards to being appealing to men. Now, the primary thing is that you are wearing clothes that suit the body of your own properly and accentuate the best assets of your own.

Now I'm not saying to head out in stripper pumps along with a nonexistent skirt which shows nearly the entire body of your own. Unless This is what you want and it can make you feel great, but do not do that since you believe it is going to make men much more attracted to you.

To be truthful, being overly skimpy to the effort of absurdity when you initially meet men really may be a turn off to some men.

The perfect way to dress is a mix of hot and leaving something on the imagination. But above all find clothing that fits the body of your own nicely and causes you to feel good.

## 9. Hair

Every man has various preferences with regards to hair and generally all that you truly have to focus on is you feel great about it.

No matter whether it is a simple, layered moderate length cut or maybe hair that is long or maybe shorter hair... The issue is you really feel great and also take the time with regards to carrying out the hair of your own.

## 10. Smell

Perfume is truly a thing that a lot of women over do. Most men don't like strong perfume. You are a lot better off sticking with something quite light and being extremely traditional with just how much you spray.

Getting really clean is clearly crucial and goes without thinking in conditions of smelling good; drenching yourself in perfume isn't. Something most men agree upon is the fact that women's hair usually smells great from all of the shampoo products as well as stuff. The issue is less is much more.

## 11. Hair "Down There"

Today this is an extremely unique preference type of scenario. You actually just have to concentrate on taking care of this particular a part of the body of your own in the terminology of hair and take action.

Until you're planning to hold all the hair of your own (rarer nowadays but once again This is a completely personal choice and there are several men that do this way therefore if there is a man who you know likes this particular go for it). I will state in general, although, trimming at the very minimum is a wise idea.

There is a great deal of debate about being totally bare or being largely bare and working with a landing strip. You are able to do a lot of various fun things with this particular. And an additional profit (in addition to men finding it hot) is basically that you are going to feel attractive realizing you're "groomed" down there. It is as much so that you can feel attractive as it's for him to discover you sexy.

A few Really Blunt (And Explicit) Tips In order to Attract The Men You would like These are going in order to be incredibly honest as well as uncensored... but are created to provide you with the raw truth and also to assist you almost as practical.

The key to most of those is that you're comfy. If you're not comfortable next there's no reason for doing these things. If you're, although, it is going to come off as extremely gorgeous. Being more comfortable is attractive.

## 12. Touch Yourself before Him and Let Him Watch

It will be incredibly hard to locate a man who doesn't find this to become an outrageous turn on. I will not actually get into this further though I believe what I stated speaks for itself. Get it done in a manner that feels comfortable for yourself and just in case it feels comfortable.

## 13. Be a Lady in a "Freak" and the Streets In the Sheets

Yes. I in fact just wrote the cliche. I cannot think I'm also writing it though it is such a succinct way for describing just about the most appealing issues to many men: a woman who is presentable along with one of the ways when she is reaching the planet behind closed doors brings away a completely different wild, sexual side.

Having the ability to really let go in the room will allow it to be even more enjoyable for each of you and him. Holding back out of anxiety about being judged as well as being awkward will simply do a disservice to each of you and him.

I realize this might not be comfy for you, but in case you are taking baby steps and find a method to get genuinely confident "letting go" you are going to notice just how much this turns men on. Do what feels natural, not everything you believe you're "supposed to do."

## 14. Create The Pleasure of your own A priority Too

This is vital. Many people are just concerned about their own pleasure and others only concerned about the opposite person's pleasure.

What is probably the most appealing way to concentrate on pleasure? Focus on both the pleasure of your own and his. Make yummy pleasure a high priority without ignoring the reality that you would like him to feel happy at the very same time.

Ignoring the pleasure of your own will do you a disservice because not merely are you going to be losing out on an outrageous level of great thoughts, though you are going to lose the chance to convert him on!!!

Most men are turned on when they are able to make women feel genuine pleasure. And don't fake it since most men are able to tell.

## 15. Tease Him

This method is a tad challenging because there's a fine line between "good" teasing which drives a man insane in a great method as well as "bad" teasing that can make men frustrated as well as irritated.

In case you're into him and really feel sexually attracted to him, allow the appeal pile up by touching him carefully throughout the interactions of your own with him.

Begin with innocent touches and be extremely nonchalant and natural once you get it done. For instance, in case you're sitting alongside one another, you can sort of inch a small little closer to him and also have the leg of your own against the leg of his and do not state a word about it, simply benefit from the second. Or maybe you could casually touch the thigh of his, like it is probably the most typical thing in the globe.

**16. Do Not Be Afraid to Be Yourself**
With regard to being appealing to men, most women are different in the terminology of what makes them exclusively appealing.

Some women tend to be more innocent along with cutesy, others are much sexier & intense, others a mix of all these... a few tend to be more outgoing and expressive, others tend to be more afraid and desire men to get control.

Some women are totally unafraid to take others and control love to be dominated. The thing is finding everything you feel confident with and understand that some men are going to be very attracted to you and these specific aspects of the personality of your own.

There's no use trying to be completely different than the way you obviously are, because This is what men find very attractive: women who's being true and genuine to herself, the desires of her and the instincts of her.

## THE BEST WAY TO ATTRACT MEN: THINGS MEN ABSOLUTELY LOVE

With regards to attracting men, it is often the little stuff you do that make the largest difference. While someone's physical appearance could cause a couple of first glances, you will find various other methods to get men to observe you and get you out there.

These ideas are not meant changing who you're. Every woman available has got the potential of attracting someone great. But learning how to work with what you've, and once to accentuate particular parts of the personality of your own, are key.

When you are new to the dating scene, or simply trying to revamp the game of your own, below are a few maneuvers men absolutely love.

## Good position.

A lot of us have bad posture, particularly working jobs that call for a lot of sitting. But just before you head out in an attempt to see someone brand new, you might wish to focus on standing up straight and mending all those hunched shoulders. It's absolutely nothing to do with level, but everything to do with trust. If perhaps the posture of your own is in check, you are nonverbally providing off the vibe that you are at ease with yourself, which men love.

## Understand your own voice.

The voice of your own is among the very first things he will end up noticing, particularly in case he hears you throughout the room talking with the friends of your own. It is vital that you have a good grasp of the way you come off in those situations (and in case it changes when you have had a number of drinks). in case you are not the loudest individual within the room of course, if you do not cut off of people's conversations to rule them, you will be a great deal a lot better in the eyes of his. Men as women who know how you can talk but additionally know the best way to truly listen.

## The capacity to communicate.

It is a huge myth that It is women that are only who appreciate chatting about their private lives - men frequently love it only that much. Until you begin with seriously individual things (which might rub him the wrong way) he will really like it in case you had taken time to question him about the favorite video game of his or maybe movie, and exactly where he grew up. Naturally, if this turned right into a full-fledged connection, he will have to question you those questions also. But by placing him in the limelight, he will realize you understand the way to begin a conversation as well as show interest in someone.

**Understanding how to carry a joke.**

Men should not be cruel or mean for you, though they might do a little gentle ribbing, particularly in case it comes to discussions about sports team preferences or maybe another thing easily arguable. Men are drawn to women with skin that is thick who can't take a laugh, but hurl one back.

**To make eye contact.**

When somebody makes eye contact with you, you understand they are keen on getting the attention of your own. When he is speaking plus you are looking right at him, he will realize you are locked into the discussion. But in case the eyes of your own are darting about, he will feel a little ignored or even worse, he is so boring you are searching for an out.

**Gently touching him.**

Perhaps even in case you are women touching men, simply realize that there will always be boundaries - and in case he recoils or feels surprised, simply back away and do not push the problem. Otherwise, a short stroke on the arm or maybe side hug is an excellent approach showing him you do not care about being near him. Plus, it is a good way for you to practically feel the power between you.

## Taking command of the circumstances.

It is a good gesture in case he buys you a drink, but men do not wish to need to do all of the effort. It has 2019, this means that gender rules are away from the table. Be assertive, and attempt to plan that very first date. Show him you are curious so he does not have dancing around the issue. Not simply will this show the confidence of your own, though he will be drawn to the reality that you are not the girl type who waits around for other people to make all of the moves.

## Know your limits.

No matter whether it is about precisely how late to remain out, or maybe the number of drinks you are able to have without getting careless, knowing the limits of your own proves you are an adult. You are not against experiencing a great time, though you are old adequate to understand that slurring the words of your own and stumbling across the dance floor is not fun. Staying out of control is not really appealing - men wish to be with a person who understands the way to deal with themselves.

**Remain optimistic.**

Irrespective of all of the negativity happening on the planet, it is nonetheless a lovely place. And, nobody is drawn to a downer who will inform you of the opposite. It is very easy to switch into a bad, self-loathing mode, though men are drawn to girls that have no issue going out and enjoying themselves even on a terrible day. With a good personality, he will likewise know he is able to lean on you in case he possibly needs a little mental support.

Apart from just attracting men, the characteristics above will help make you a lot better as a general man. Confidence could be your greatest asset when it is about getting ahead or even meeting someone new.

## THE BEST WAY TO SEDUCE A MAN

"It's intriguing we connect seduction with sex, when in reality, genuine seduction is the complete opposite of sex. Sex happens when want is met. Seduction isn't about the culmination or maybe gratification of desire, it's all about the thrill of the drive itself. It's the game which is played when the motivation comes closer, and also better, and closer, and also having the ability to keep that stress of wanting for a very long, long time."

Seduction is all about making him would like you, not always permitting him have you.

You can seduce men you have never ever kissed...

And also you are able to seduce men you have been with for a long time.

In either case, these strategies for how you can attract men will are available in handy.

## Seduction Tip one: Let The Your Eyes Do the Work

Want to learn how to attract a? Give him the sexy eyes of your own.
Your eyes tell him everything about just how you think. They're, actually, your biggest weapon with regards to earning the seduction war.

Here is a fascinating study: a psychologist brought together many women and men who would certainly not met before and also asked them to explore each other 's eyes for 2 minutes without saying a word.

What would you picture happened? Afterward, the vast majority of participants felt very attracted to the test partner of theirs. Among the couples actually got married a year later! This simply goes to show the strength of eye contact.

When you are speaking with a man you are attracted to, you may get anxious and flit the eyes of your own available, though you are a lot better off looking him straight in the eyes (while smiling!) while you speak or even listen. Mix up your expression according to what he is thinking. You are able to generate an eyebrow to show you do not trust him (in a playful way), as well as wink at him. You will find therefore a number of ways you are able to express yourself with the eyes of your own, so experiment and find out what gets a response.

You are able to additionally earn extended eye contact with him across a crowded room up until he takes notice, then lookout. You have hooked him, however it looks like there is something much more fascinating that has taken the attention of your own. This can pique the interest of his since he wants the attention of your own back on him, and he will walk over.

**Seduction Tip two: Practice The Dozens of your Smiles Did you understand you will find various types of smiles? Some you will not wish to use, similar to the fake smile, though you are able to continue to mix it up.**

Consider using a sly grin that states I understand one thing you do not know, mixed with a peaceful chuckle, to keep him curious about what you are wondering.

Smile truly as he approaches and says something interesting.

Try giving him a smirk in case he relies on a cheesy pickup line. You do not want to send him out with the tail of his between the legs of his, though you do want him to find out you are onto him.

Make up the own smiles of your own! Just like eye expressions, you can find a lot of solutions to use this in case you are learning how you can attract men.

**Seduction Tip three: Use Body Language**

When you are on a date or simply speaking with a man you wish to attract, be keenly conscious of the body positioning of your own. If the arms of your own are crossed or you are facing separate from him, he will not get the sense that you are interested. On the flip side, in case you lean in together with your arms propped on the dinner table or maybe your hip informs him you are open.

And never underestimate the strength of a great hair flip! Hair, especially very long hair that is loose, is especially gorgeous to most men. And so remind him of how Pantene worthy yours is.

**Seduction Tip four: Touch Him Often Touch goes hand in hand with body language. The more regularly you feel him - and we are not talking apparent caresses with these - the more he will want to touch you too. Touch reminds men of - yep, you guessed it - sex, therefore it is a subtle way of thinking I would like you.**

When you would like to learn how to attract a men with contact, concentrate on resting the fingers of your own on the forearm of his, carefully squeezing the biceps of his (oh my! what large muscles you have!), or perhaps laying the hand of your own on the shoulder of his or even back. Try it out and see in case he reciprocates inside a couple of minutes.

**Seduction Tip five: Send Seductive Texts The key to realizing how you can attract men is acknowledging that not every seduction occurs in an individual. You are able to likewise fascinate him by text. The key element here's not in order to be blatantly sexual but to utilize innuendo to get him thinking hot without pushing for it.**

Try leaving a lot of blanks for him to pack in.

I'd a dream about you survive night...
Would you know what I would do when you are here?
I am still considering that great kiss. Wow!

Actually watch that line between sex and seduction because some men are just too pleased to begin sending dick pics or maybe sexting, and that's not the goal of your own. You wish to develop anticipation, whether that is to look at you once again, kiss for at first chance, yes, or even, have sex.

**Seduction Tip six: Display Your Confidence Nothing is far more appealing compared to a confident woman.**

There is a reason I am constantly encouraging you to be confident: men love it. When you appear as you are not determined, you would likely take or even leave talking to a fellow, the desire of his to chase you kicks in.

A confident woman knows she is smart, funny, and attractive. She does not require men to express to her that. In reality, she does not require a man at all. And nothing makes men need a woman much more than when she shows she does not require him but needs him. Thus own which.

In case he compliments you, laugh and appear in the eyes of his and say thank you. And Better yet, I realize!

Keep the shoulders of your own back. Shoulders forward state you are insecure. The opposite states you own the space.

Put on apparel that flatters you. You do not have to put on very short dresses or plunging necklines being attractive, but do don clothes that say I am aware I look fab.

**Seduction Tip seven: Show Off The Intellectual Side of your own If you are thinking you have to play down the smarts of your own to learn how you can seduce a man, you are wrong. Most men, particularly sapiosexuals - also referred to as nymphomaniacs - get switched on by intelligence. In case you understand you are smarter than a rocket scientist, then allow it to show!**

Note: there is a fine line between showing off the intellectual side of your own and also simply being a know-it-all. in case you are attempting to attract men, you are able to discuss books you have checked out and items you are keen on, but do not begin correcting him in case he states something wrong.

Him: ...you understand, since the sunshine revolves around the Earth...

You: Actually...

Nothing is going to kill a men's libido quicker than being corrected. Therefore simply leave it.

This is especially beneficial in case you see a fellow by way of a dating app since you frequently have some terrific meat about what he is into. If you notice an ebook or maybe subject he is keen on his dating profile, carry it up. The far more obscure, the greater. He will be blown away you have any idea about it! (Just make certain you really do).

**Seduction Tip eight: Be slightly Hot as well as Cold**

I know a lot of women who think the way to seduce a man is throwing themselves at him. Exactly how will he realize you need him in case you are not draped all over him?

In reality, the alternative holds true.
The woman is not a challenge. The woman he'll chase is one which pours all the attention of her on him...then excuses herself to obtain a drink or even say hi to a buddy. The women who once he shows interest, back off a bit.

Should you discover you have been performing a lot of touching or eye batting, pull back and also let him step up the game of his to teach you he is engaged.

**Seduction Tip nine: Let the Dance Floor Perform the Seducing Make the moves of your own on the dance floor.**

Dancing is a fantastic way to show the attraction of your own without requiring any witty discussion. And no, there is no twerking for you!

Assuming you have been making eyes at men throughout the room and also you believe he is serious though he has not yet produced a move, sashay over to him, grab the hand of his, then pull him away on the dance floor. You are able to get close, but there is no grinding essential. Simply having you inside such close proximity is going to work the magic of its. Try letting your hips loosen, smile to indicate you are getting a great time, and throw the hands of your own over the shoulders of his.

When you have not yet danced with him, get available on your own and dance while you watch him. can make it kind of obvious you want he was there along with you on the dance floor!

**Seduction Tip ten: Have Some Deliberate "Accidents" If you are sitting at a table next to this particular man, allow your leg to clean them several times of his. He will question, was that a crash?**

Drop something and get it so you show off the body of your own. Or lower it so that your fingers collide as he additionally reaches to get it.

He is going to think these small gestures are accidents, though he will still be seduced and would like you more.

While several of these hints regarding how to attract men want you to obtain just a little out of the comfort zone of your own, generally speaking, you need to feel at ease performing them (if not, skip that one). I 100 % believe you've to be yourself to be able to seduce men. Or else, you come off as inauthentic, and he will see through you.

If you are confident and sexy, you will prove yourself to be real. He will like you, body, mind, and soul in case he views you understand who you're and also what you would like (including him!).

You may have to practice these tips regarding how to seduce a man so you perform them confidently and flawlessly. Imagine every day you go on being the chance to perform. Take emotional notes on what have very best outcomes (hair flip coupled with a gentle touch on the wrist? Check!) so you know using it the next time.

Even though seduction is not related to sex, it is a fantastic lead up to it in case you wish to have sex with a fellow you are discovering. Keep in mind that fear is fifty percent the fun, and so let that sexual tension actually increase therefore whenever you do finally choose to enter into bed with this particular man, it blows the mind of his completely. Take the time of your own, however. While the seduction efforts of your own might make him even more willing to voice your actual physical relationship together, you additionally have to remain on the exact same page for doing it to happen. When it is correct, it will happen.

# WHAT MEN WANT IN BED: WAYS TO PUSH HIM WILD

Indeed, we are all aware men love getting blow tasks, fantasize about threesomes, moreover commonly really love sex and need it all of the time. But we need to delve in a bit deeper into what men really would like in bed and wish women knew.

## 1. It is About The Attitude

Men wish to have sex with a woman who's really to it. Eagerness as well as enthusiasm go quite a distance. A lot of women hold the mindset which simply letting men have sex with her is some gift type, along with men detest that.

In case you're simply starting the motions, and performing it from obligation, as a favor, or even since you would like anything in exchange, that is a significant turn-off.

The best turn onto a man has been with women who are experiencing the sex simply almost as he's.

## 2. Make Him Feel Wanted

Men possess a deep need to be sexually desired. Simply telling men "I want you" is able to do all sorts of things for the ego of his.

Letting him know exactly how much you like sex with him additionally works great. Experiment with informing him, "I like having you inside me." If you are way too afraid to state that aloud, test texting him.

When you do not wish to be that direct, you are able to make him get you looking at the butt of his or maybe some additional component of the body of his which turns you on. Maybe even touch him over usual, particularly in naughty places.

Objectify him a small, lust after him, and let him know exactly how much he turns you on. You will catch him unawares and make him think as he is gorgeous you cannot handle yourself.

## 3. Initiate Once In a While

Traditionally, men are the people who initiate sex. They are wired in that way as an outcome of the ancient hunter ancestors of theirs.

Most men love to take charge and therefore are cool with initiating sex the majority of the time. Though it is able to get old when he's to become the one to get it done every time.

Recall how men have to feel wanted? Once you never ever initiate sex, the man of your own may begin to feel as you are not drawn to him.

Whisper in the ear of his how badly you need him inside you, or maybe stick you hand down the pants of his. In case you want to rock the world of his, wake him with a morning BJ.

Nevertheless, you choose to initiate sex, it is guaranteed to make the men of your own happiness because after he does not need to be the one to get it done.

## 4. Take Control

Even though men like to be in control, they love to be dominated every sometimes also. It is able to get boring after some time to be the person who's constantly in control.

It moves men crazy when a women grab him, pushes him down, and also has the way of her with him. A woman who knows what she desires as well as goes after it's an enormous turn-on.

When you have a tendency to allow your men to take control at all times, consider turning the tables and also taking the reins sometimes. Not merely will your man stay in for a surprise, though he will know without a doubt just how much you would like him.

## 5. Confidence Is actually Key

Confidence is definitely the sexiest trait a woman is able to have. Whatever insecurities you've, recall that the man of your own is along with you since he is drawn to you and also would like to have sex with you.

A woman who could get the clothes of her off with self-confidence is a lot more appealing compared to a woman that asks the man of her to switch the lights off initially. Men are visual creatures for off on seeing you in all the naked glory of your own.

In case you're uncomfortable, try smooth lighting which will conceal some flaws you are stressing over. But in all probability men wouldn't notice those small jiggles or even that cellulite you are so concerned with. They are so thrilled to be there along with you, naked!

## 6. Be Vocal

Men love it if you let loose for loud. A woman who could express herself in the room is an enormous turn-on.

No matter whether it's moaning as well as groaning or even uninhibited screaming, they recognize the feedback that however much they are engaging in is working. Men have to find out they are doing an excellent job. They wish to find out they are traveling you very wild you cannot help but scream in ecstasy.

Toss in a bit of dirty talk also, you will send him over the edge! Try giving him a filthy play-by-play or even let him know what you would like to do to him following.

## 7. Give Instructions

Every woman is different when it is in regard to what they like. Men appreciate just a little guidance regarding how to pleasure you, or else it is a great deal of error and trial on the part of theirs.

You're the one individual that knows precisely what it requires for getting you off, so support men out there and give him a few guidelines to direct him in the correct path. Do not be afraid about it!

Regardless if you direct him with words or sounds of encouragement when he is on the proper track, or perhaps flat out tell him what you should do when he is not, most men will likely be thankful. If you would like extra points, get a bit of dirty when you are telling him what you would like him to do for you.

A woman that has learned what she desires is a turn on. Additionally, men obtain a great deal of sexual gratification from pleasing their partners. Whatever you are able to do to assist him to amuse you is a win for both of you.

**8. Worship Him**

For men, sex is a lot about feeding their egos. They wish to really feel desired, appreciated, and worshipped.

And This is why oral sex is very important to men. They're fixated on it a great deal because they need you to worship the cocks of theirs simply almost as they do.

The key element to giving a mind-blowing BJ is really enjoying it. Keeping the energy to send out the man of your own with the advantage with a knee-buckling, thigh quivering orgasm can allow you to feel attractive as hell.

Make eye contact with the man of your own and let him see exactly how much pleasure it offers you to please him. You will make him feel like a rock star!

## 9. Be Adventurous

Men like women that are ready to accept trying things that are new in the bedroom. Everybody has a unique sexual appetite, that be willing and adventurous to test new flavors. It is boring to perform the very same thing on a regular basis anyway.

It is likewise crucial not to create men feel terrible about anything he really wants to do. When you are ready to accept the fantasies of his, he will really feel risk-free to express himself sexually & associated with you on a greater level.

If you are not at ease with whatever it's he really wants to do, that is good. Simply do not judge him for doing it or make him think like a pervert. Negotiate as well as attempt to locate something which works for each of you.

## 10. Do not Fake It

Women generally mean perfectly whenever they fake an orgasm. They do not wish to bruise their men's ego so that they simply let him believe he finished the task.

Nevertheless, you are really giving positive reinforcement for something which did not work. If perhaps the man of your own is not pleasing you, tell him exactly how he is able to. Above most, the man of your own truly does need to please you plus faking it does not permit him to function as the most effective lover he is able to be.

If you know you are not going to come and you're prepared to finish, you are able to simply tell him. An immediate teaching such as, "I prefer you to come now," is going to let him realize he is totally free to allow himself go without stressing about whether it has been long enough for you.

## THINGS YOU COULD DO WITH YOUR MOUTH WHICH WILL DRIVE A MAN CRAZY

Clearly, you know the way to make the partner of your own feel great in the bedroom. But in case you are attempting to mix things up a provide a surprise to the partner of your own, did you understand there is a great deal you are able to do without needing to go full-on 50 Shades? The best part is, you've everything you need actually. It 's...your mouth.

## 1. Focus on His Ears

...But no importance to go nuts. The ear is able to get subtle sensations - and a reduced amount of is much more. Here is what you should do: Place the lips of your own an inch away from the ear of his and launch a gradual sigh. Next, then take his earlobe between the lips of your own and gently tug. This can pull at, and indirectly stimulate, the nerve endings within the ear. "These nerves are rarely activated, therefore you will really blow his mind whenever you do this". Thus, yes: ears are usually an erogenous zone!

## 2. Do not forget his Fingers

If you believe kisses on the hand are just for men courting women in the 1940s, then you have not tried this one: Place the idea of the tongue of your own on the webbed location in the foundation of the fingers of his, and then gradually glide the way of your own up the edge. This particular move is going to give him goose bumps because this particular place is extremely sensitive - but, similar to the nerves of the inner ear of his, it seldom gets a lot of focus. Next, making him totally outrageous, walk up the idea of his finger between your lips. "It's suggestive of what I might be doing down below".

## 3. Kiss the Roof of his Mouth

Which means you figure you have explored every inch of the mouth of his with yours? The fact is, the main subject that is frequently ignored is the top of the mouth of his, which is among the most ticklish areas of the entire body, claims Hess. And so the next time you are lip-to-lip, flick the tongue of your own twice or once in an arc along this particular region (any more may send him right into a match of giggles). Katrina, thirty-three, has discovered this move works wonders on her husband. "When folks kiss, they often aim for the tongue," she says. "But the very first time I ran the tongue of mine across the top of my husband's mouth, he was like,' Whoa!' Now I realize that in case I actually wish to get an increase from him, that is what I have to do."

## 4. Tease Him
Lightly graze the lips of your own (keeping them as become dry) that is possible throughout the forehead of his, looping gradually over to his temple after which right down to the mouth of his. This dried out brush, as Hess calls it, is going to have a different experience from the normal damp kiss. That is since the facial skin is included with almost invisible fuzz known as vellum hairs. A small, slight touch is going to activate these hairs, inducing sublime shivers.

The sweetness of the kiss will even improve your emotional connections to each other. "It's tender but gorgeous, which often tends to make men smile". Meaning a kiss this way says, "Let's have it on" and "I like you."

## 5. Notice his Neck
Not many kisses establish an I-want-you-now link as people on the neck. In order to use the enthusiasm level up a notch,

carefully pull the head of his again and on the edge, which could present an extra-sensitive tendon operating out of the ear on the shoulder. Beginning in the foundation of the ear of his, work the way of your own down the ridge, arbitrarily alternating between gentle kisses and small nibbles and so he will not understand what is coming next.

## 6. Try an innovative Sensitive Spot

The underside of the tongue of your own is going to feel truly great on his most vulnerable spots - namely the nipples of his, a frequently ignored erogenous zone on men. The silky texture of its is going to feel gorgeous in his most vulnerable places - specifically the nipples of his, a frequently ignored erogenous zone on men. "Although numerous men are ashamed to point out it - since it appears as a thing exclusively women must want - they secretly crave having you focus on this particular area".

Consequently flick the bottom section of the tongue of your own from side to side throughout these sweet places. Next, as he gets into it, toss the senses of his for a loop by changing to the rougher, top side of the tongue of your own, alternating again & forth. "Nerves often go numb whenever they get exactly the same kind of stimulation for way too long". But if you change from a single texture type to the next, you will have the senses of his on optimum alert - that will keep him begging for a lot more.

## 7. Kiss his Thigh
Starting right above the knee of his, grow a light-as-a-feather kiss there, then work the way of your own up, raising the stress of the lips of your own on the skin of his the farther you go.

## 8. Play With Temperature
Everything you will need is a cup of espresso or maybe an iced drink because of this technique. Have a sip, then press your warm (or maybe cold) mouth to the inner wrist of his, growing small kisses up the interior of his arm. "The veins are near the surface area in this specific region, and this helps make it particularly open to touch".

Plus, you will be stimulating both temperatures- as well as pressure-sensitive nerves, creating a complete brand new dimension of sensations.

## 9. Kiss his Stomach

Involving your men's navel and the nether region of his is a strip of hairstyle referred to as the "treasure trail," so named due to the sensitivity of its (not to point out the reality it leads right where he is dying for you personally to go). Want to show him precisely how prize-worthy this trail is really? Starting right beneath the navel of his, take some strands of hair in between the lips of your own and take - just tough a sufficient amount of he is able to think it, but carefully a sufficient amount of that he is not jumping from the skin of his. The pinpricks of small pain you will produce will send out jolts of electrical power through the lower abdominal region of his, as well as register below the belt.

"Light locks pulling indirectly activates nerves deep below the skin 's surface, and that is one thing straight skin-to-skin contact cannot do". Additionally, the downward path you are proceeding in is going to make your men's imagination run wild with hot' n' heavy choices.

## 10. Give a Hands-Free Massage

Straddle the husband of your own as he lies on the stomach of his, and then press the mouth of your own securely into the nape of the neck of his. With the tongue of your own flexed so it is pointy, probe the grooves on each side of the vertebrae of his, gradually working the way of your own down to his tailbone. "Essentially you are providing him a shiatsu massage using your tongue rather than the fingers" of your own. When massages often lull him to sleep, do not be shocked if perhaps this has rather the complete opposite effect. If you use the lips of your own rather than the hands of your own, the massage of your own immediately moves from relaxing to racy.

## 11. Make your Mouth Vibrate

Here is one you may not have thought of: humming. To start with you may think a little strange, though the payoff is going to be well worth it. "Humming causes the mouth of your own to vibrate in a manner that feels much like sex toys". Additionally, varying the pitch of the voice of your own causes a selection of sensations: Lower pitches produce reduced vibrations; higher pitches, quicker ones.

## 12. Take note of the Knees

"This area is among the most underrated erogenous zones. "The knees are loaded with nerve endings; that is exactly why individuals are usually ticklish there". The backs of the knee are particularly vulnerable, since the nervous feelings are around the counter, she provides. For optimum sensual influence, swivel the tongue of your own across the crease after which blow on the spot. This particular puff of air is going to cause the fluid to evaporate, creating a thrilling hot-then-cold sensation. Additionally, he will have the ability to truly believe you breathe, that is going to tune the body of his into yours and give the intimacy of your own a surcharge.

## 13. Suck on the Bottom of his Lips

Take only the bottom lip of his involving yours and draw on it carefully, that will provide far more blood on the surface area of the skin of his, thus, making this place more delicate. In order to get him in on the action, have him suck on the top lip of your own while you are focusing on the bottom of his one; afterward switch. "A lot of men know just 2 kisses: the lip kiss and also the French kiss". "This is something totally different, and also because you are able to change roles, it never becomes monotonous."

## 14. Tickle his Torso

Although "they will not readily admit it," there are scores of locations men will really like in the event that you lavished interest on. Flicking the tongue of your own across noted erogenous zones - just like the underarm - plus not-so-expected places, like the rib cage of his.

## 15. Present New Sensations

There is far more to the mouth of your own than merely a tongue. "You've had a tongue, mouth, and even teeth". "All 3 present an alternative feel." In between licking as well as sucking very sensitive zones including the nipples of his, try out grazing them with the teeth of your own for a bit of added excitement.

## 16. Begin Talking

It does not get any less complicated than this. While sighs and moans are hot in their own right, whispering phrases, needs, or perhaps simply the name of theirs is such a turn on. Bonus: Getting vocal about what you would like him to complete for you promises you will both appreciate one another more.

## 17. Call Him Up

Sexting is fun and just, though nothing beats good old-fashioned telephone sex when you are much apart. Use this chance to refer to your dirtiest fantasies to one another, and do not forget the toys.

## 18. Get it Back

"Have him lie on his stomach, and then gradually trace a zig-zag up the spine of his, beginning from the really bottom". "The spine has plenty of nerve endings, therefore you will have him begging for more."

## 19. Test out Other areas of his Body

Did you know that you will find a lot more hot places you can touch the partner of your own? And when all those places you feel him feel great, consider just how much better he will think when the mouth of your own is on it. Merely a number of places to consider: the elbows of his, the toes of his, the clavicle of his,.. you receive the concept. Every man differs and will have various specific turn-ons, so it is really worth trying newer spots.

## 20. Question What He would Like - And Tell Him Everything you Want

Indeed, questions may be sexy - though the answers could be a lot better. Ask him if there is something he would like so that you can try, whether it is right now or down the road. And make certain you inform him what you wish to see - he will be much more than pleased to oblige.

# THE BEST WAY TO SEDUCE A MEN WITH WORDS

## FLIRTING

Newsflash! Generally there simply are not sensational phrases or maybe brilliant lines which are planning to cause men to fall head over heels crazy about you, sorry. But what you are able to do is attempt to be playful also publicly suggestive with them.

In case you tell him what you're thinking straight up, that is a risky move since you are possibly going to guess right along with nail it or maybe you will send him running fast and far.

You are more or less safe with some just nonaggressive flirting that is going to let him realize you would like to get it to the subsequent level, though you are not going to pressure him a lot of to deliver.

The very last thing you should do is provide him stage fright!

## Feed Him Sincere Compliments

You may think men are not keen on hearing about precisely how handsome they're, though you could not be much more wrong according to the pros.

Think over it for a minute.

Everyone likes a compliment again and now if it is sincere correct?

Plus there's a distinction between sweet nothings a man informs women and what she provides to him. Take the mushy gushy out of the compliment of your own and you are on the proper track.
Lastly, regardless of what you do, see to it that you're complimenting him with fact. In case he senses you're merely attempting to pour him up, then you definitely may get yourself into a bit of warm water.

Have a Keen Interest in the life of his - Daily And Otherwise It is crucial that you are taking a genuine interest in his life in case you're likely to attempt to seduce men with the words of your own. Ensure you're listening to what he claims & do not hesitate to mirror or even replicate the words he's thinking back.

This simply lets him realize he is simply not blowing smoke while the mind of your own is everywhere else.
When a man knows a woman is listening, he is going to open the door to seduction when you play the cards of your own right.

Of course, the option is yours.

## Don't Hesitate To Play With Your Words

Of course everyone appears to like words of praise however when you're attempting to seduce men with words, you might like to try challenging him a bit. But just in case you have received the backbone for it.

If the seduction tactics of your own are not working extremely well, take a step back and try to be a bit more distant.

Challenge the thoughts of his with the contrary and discover how he responds. Do not get negative or aggressive too here or maybe you will wind up looking like a dork. Leave him hanging a little but informing him of a story and also telling him you will end it later.

You won't ever know until you attempt, right?

## Strong Isn't Always Bad

When everything else fails, you might have to take out the huge guns and also be immediate with him. Explain to him you do not truly care what you do tonight though you need to do it with him.

Truth - This is a bit of risk but on the other hand, it is advisable to figure it out sooner instead of later on.

## Try Leaving A Lasting First Impression

We have all made mistakes judging individuals by the first impression but that appears to be the default of human nature. So it is essential that you simply make specific you leave a perfectly great first impression with men. Especially the people you're trying to seduce.

Psychologically speaking, you're on the proper track in case you give him a great first impression.

Show him you're secure and confident in yourself and you're happy and light-hearted. Men simply do not want to get into emotional craziness and drama if they are able to help it.

Attempt to ensure the conversation flows and get the questions that are going to get him opening and talking up a little. Also, whenever you get him talking, you're not as likely to screw up!

## Work With Your Eyes Seduce Him

You will discover not many things the eyes are able to conceal when you have got the sunglasses of your own off and This is one thing you're likely to need to make use of.

In the real picture, when you're trying to attract men with words, it is the eyes of your own who are gonna nail it. If you make eye contact with men, you're showing him you are interested and curious. Talk about an excellent beginning.

Eyes cause emotion and they actually are completely gorgeous.

Hold your gaze for over a second and do not hesitate to bashfully look away occasionally. Do not stare but let him realize you're looking at him and wish to keep on searching for all of the right reasons.

When you toss in a sexy smile or 2 as soon as your glances cross, you're providing him a lot more signals that you're thinking about seducing him.

Do not forget, you have to be entirely slight with this method because in case you do not, it is going to backfire as well as feel phony or pressed, just not sensuously gorgeous.

## Straight Up Seduction With The Words Of your own

Most everyone loves a great conversation so long as it is not only one-sided. Both men and gals wish to be heard but are not thinking about doing all of the talking.

If you pay attention to what a man is thinking and in addition help the conversation, you're informing him straight up you wish to know much more. So when you wish to know a lot more in regards to men, it is safe to state the door is ready to accept the subsequent level in case it comes to which.

At this moment you are not planning to get a man to fall in love with you by speaking with him, but in case you're running a good conversation with men, you're informing him you're curious.

Be positive with the words of your own and show him you're not hesitant to start a little. And certainly do not pull out the judgment card of your own in any way, form or shape. You may actually wish to step outside your comfort zone a bit and playfully tease him and ask him a question that crosses the buddy line a small.

It will not take you long to be an expert in reading through a men demeanor and then proceeding accordingly. Maintain the eye contact going during the conversation of your own to let him know you're listening as well as fixated with him.

## Simply Be the Main And Just You

In case you're experiencing both anxious and nervous while attempting to attract men with words, it is alright showing him this or even Better yet explain to him.

He is along with you for a reason. Consider that for a second.

## Savor The Moment

One of the more sexy things regarding women happens when she's smiling and enjoying themselves. So stop the negative moods and do not sulk if you do not get everything you want.

Get creative and enjoy yourself with the words of your own. Add just a little effort and time into the seduction progression and he is going to appreciate it.

What in case he does not?
Kick his sorry butt to the curb and move on.
Simply Ask Him
This one seems a bit too obvious but if you truly desire to seduce men with words, simply ask him what he really wants to hear. Often directly to the stage works wonders.

## Chill On The Cheesy Stuff

You are going to fail when you attempt to attract men while pretending to become a slutty porn star. Remember to knock that one off before you begin. It is not what he wants, he wants hard.

Whenever you tone it down a notch or perhaps 2 and show him you're becoming totally honest, that is obviously sexy.

What about attempting the subtle course to seduce men with words?

## Slight Tricks To Seduce A Men Over The Phone

In case you want to record the interest of the men species, you're much better to dress up hot in a warm costume than begin a strong mental discussion. Nevertheless, it's possible to create men fall for you with only words, but you have got to know what you are doing.

Here is how you can seduce men mildly over text using simply words - Magical.

Taking Action In order to Seduce A men Via Text Messages:

This particular strategy is particularly effective in case you're already friends with the men or even have no less than met presently. Allow me to share the suggestions that are going to assist you with the focus of your own of seducing men with words.

## Simply Tell Him Plain As Day That You're Considering Him

Every man loves to hear the woman he's keen on is thinking of them.

to provide you with more bang for the buck of your own, be sure you use a lot of sweet emojis
This works great things on him mentally.

Use The Name Of His Repeatedly When You're Texting Him Back And Forth

What this does is make the texting of your own unique and personalized, which does not get a lot superior to that!

## Save The Dirty Texting For Later

Do not cross the line and begin with unclean texts. You could be subtle and gentle by confessing to him you simply got from the bath or maybe something around the lines. Try giving him the door to believe soiled but do not communicate it.

## Keep Him Wondering With A Small Amount Of Mystery

Don't provide him all of the details because that is going getting him bored fast. So hold the explanations short & sweet so he will keep wanting a lot more.

shoot the text message during the night if at all possible and make certain you are not showing him your full hand
Let the imagination of his do the job for him. A good course to seducing men.
Before you can get way too carried away, below are a few set rules for seducing men with words.

If you believe using just one of those strategies will get him, you're dead wrong. It is going to carry a bit of trial and time and error. Be patient and persistent consistently.

No one rule fits everybody so you have to be skeptical of exactly how a man reacts to the seduction tactics of your own. If you're with men in which the synergy between the 2 of you simply takes off from the beginning, and then just about any seduction method works.

Along with other men, there might simply be one route to attract him and yes it usually takes oodles of time, you simply never know.

*If you're trying to attract him for the long term, steady and slow then will win the race. Do not allow it to be way too obvious but be chronic whenever you have to, confidently chronic.

Indeed, physical touch and intimacy are vitally important in any romantic relationship though it is not everything. It is a bit of challenging however when you're first getting to know a man, you are able to seduce him with words to start your own online business.

It is a bit less risky than the bodily material for sure.

With regard to seducing men with words, there's no simple answer. It is everything about experimentation and calculated error and trial. Figure out what authority techniques work for yourself and go because of it.

## HOT SPOTS ON A MEN'S BODY YOU HAVE TO DEFINITELY KNOW ABOUT

Everyone loves sex, right? There's no wondering that. But connecting with an old or new partner might be, very well, too much to handle at times. At this time you will find plenty of places of one's body to relish in the minutes you're getting right down to business.

While you are able to argue that any zone on a dude's body may be an erogenous zone if treated correctly, you are going to find several unique locations that are a lot finer when compared with others.

## 1. His Hair

Do you identify precisely how wonderful it feels when someone plays with the locks of your own? Exact same for men, gals. Men have nerve endings on the scalp of theirs that are linked to the vast majority of the body of theirs, once the locks of theirs are meticulously pulled when they are kissed and even stored, it sends stimulation to the majority of the body of theirs.

Fix this: While kissing, think about running the recommendations of the toes of your own through the locks of his, with the head of his thoroughly, consequently a bit harder by using a tug. Just in case he responds with moderate pleasure and appears moans, pull harder, then let go right before he wants you to. This playful tease with drive him legitimate outrageous.

## 2. His Toes

Shrimpin' anyone? Certainly, this is what it's widely known as in case you draw on your own partner's toes (or perhaps they really do to you.) This is extremely erotic mainly because foot definitely is a nonconventional hotbed of sensation just awaiting many stimulations.

Fix this: During warm foreplay, shift the kisses of your own teasingly down the entire body of his in place unless you're all the way down at the feet of his. Draw on your partner's toes - additionally, on occasion actually lick the bottom portion of the feet arch of theirs. Just probably have him use a shower before, mmk?

## 3. The Feet in General

Besides merely feeling great, there's a great reason reflexology massages are very popular. You can find loads of nerve endings in the feet, that makes for a great spot to promote.

Fix this: Don't care, you don't have to become a foot fetishist to ace this. Begin through the use of many massage oil and rubbing the foot of his - especially the arch of the foot. When you'd love to put in a bit of tongue and kisses into the mix, do the. Then swap roles and permit it to become the turn of your own.

## 4. The Prostate

Introducing: Most likely the most underrated part of many men 's bodies. The prostate gland is a huge erogenous zone of men. If correctly stimulated, this may bring extreme pleasure to the men of your own. Ladies, this is essentially the men 's G spot and it's more sensitive.

Fix this: Run a lubricated finger at the anus of his to begin. This particular stimulation by itself may be adequate for him, but if he's down for much more, after the muscle groups have had a chance to loosen up, put in the index finger of your own approximately 2 inches inside - where you should stay in a place to feel the prostate of his. Bend the finger of your own up towards his abdomen and stroke it.

## 5. His Imagination

Fine, so maybe This is not really a concrete item you're competent to touch? but in defense of mine, you're in a position to surely nevertheless cause this specific facet of him. Try letting him have some time to think about the touch of your own in front of your hands turn up on the skin of his. The most effective tease.

Fix this: Whisper in the ear of his softly and explain to him the things you are more likely to do to him without touching a hair on the entire body of his. Little idea WTF to recommend? Just pretend as you're sexting in addition to point out the points to him IRL.

## 6. His Butt Cheek

Ah, the sweet spot of the bod. He's gonna be vulnerable with these. To strike the butt cheek of his, dull carefully, is apt to advertise the whole region. Think of it the same as a slow vibration streaming throughout the insides of his.

Fix this: If the boy of your own is prepared to take a bit of spanky play, this is incredible to undertake while he's additionally for you in almost any deviation of missionary. Squeeze the booty of his when he's striking just the ideal area, or perhaps get him a fast spank if you're both into it. Don't wait to grab or stroke there.

## 7. The Philtrum

The philtrum, or perhaps small groove above the mouth of your own, is certainly considered an erogenous zone. In truth, she talks about, the word itself, philtrum, translates from the Latin phrase for love potion.

Fix this: To promote the philtrum of his, grow an incredibly gentle kiss on this specific area, right before operating the tongue of your own down the groove to satisfy top of the lip of his.

## 8. The Raphe

The raphe stands apart as the dividing line that runs all over the middle of the genitalia of his from the anus on the purpose of the penis of his, complete with the perineum, scrotum, and shaft.

Fix this: Use the tongue of your own to trace over the sequence and also teasing him into the jaws of your own. To be able to shoot things a stride a lot more, choose a lubed up bullet vibrator like the We-Vibe Tango, to trace on the series too, while you inhale, lick, then simply suck together with the vibrator.

## 9. Inner Thigh

The inner thigh is quite close to the penis, despite having no sensation of touch, merely being in that school will definitely get him anticipating what's next.

Fix this: Take time off your own to kiss and lick the internal thigh of his prior to heading to touch the penis of his when performing oral. Tease him & play around with the mouth of your own. You're competent going from mild fluttering kisses to harder sucking.

## 10. Outsole Lips

Lips on the entire are only about probably the most susceptible parts of the body. Take the time of your own while kissing - there are cause nibbling and deviation of anxiety can help you over the edge when performed accurately.

Fix this: Nibble the bottom mouth area of theirs & possibly even going for the tougher bite (in case they seem to be ready to accept it). The sensations of living out of a tender kiss too many teeth will shock the men of your own and trigger the mind of his.

## 11. All those V-Lines

Aside from getting enjoyable and sexy you are able to check out, the V zone is a good foundation of enjoyment for the partner of your own. Not simply may it be a turn-on he gets front row tickets to open you promote him, although it's a pit stop producing on the way to bone town.

Fix this: Have his site on the rear of his when you straddle him as well as offer him what he truly wants: a viewpoint of the head of your own whenever you create the means of your own down on him. Beginning from the belly button of his, work with your fingers and nails to trace a line down out of the lucky trail of his stopping before you hit total groin. Then, retrace the steps of your own, but make use of the tongue of your own to trace a V shape coming from the hips of his to directly above the penis of his. Draw it out and genuinely tease him until he can't obtain it any longer.

## 12. The outside of His Lower Lip

You are aware that area in between the lower lip of your own as well as the face of your own exactly where you usually break out? Yeah, the individual that a private hair generally sprouts out of? That's an erogenous zone! This tiny, fine curve is really loaded with extra sensitive nerve receptors.

Fix this: Suck the lower lip of his in the mouth of your own the next time you're generating- Positive Many Meanings - also and away use the thought of the tongue of your own to stroke this specific below lip area. The motions trigger the whole erogenous zone in a teasing fashion, which will put him on the erotic advantage. And by keeping the lower lip of his inside yours, you magnify the sensation. It'll actually feel like electronically powered currents are recording out of the jaws of his straight on the part of his.

## 13. The Front of his Neck

I believe you've never thought of your dude's Adam's apple as an erogenous zone, huh? Just in case you have, congrats, you have to probably be writing it instead of me. But simply for the normies nowadays, the idea powering this will come out of the manner the thyroid (just below Adam's apple) is clearly attached to the sex organs, based on first Chinese medicine.

Fix this: Give him a throat perform - very little, not in that way, (you can to re hinge your jaw now.) Have him lie on the rear of his and nearly simply bring his Adam's apple. Maintain the tongue of your own dull in addition to light, not in excess of pressure! Massage the location with wide circular motions to ensure you're hitting that T area of the thyroid.

## 14. His Nipples

While men nipples are essentially precisely the just like women nipples, they might be a bit finer compared to yours since men aren't used that will get them touched so frequently. For a good deal of men, the nipples of theirs are uncharted territory - an erogenous zone they haven't experimented with. Touch them, nevertheless, as well as you are going to send out shock waves of pleasure radiating through him, she offers.

Fix this: Britton suggests having him lie on the rear of his plus continuously licking out of the areola of his inward, not unlike an ice cream cone but seldom touching tongue to nip. Get better and also closer before you flick the nipple of his with the tongue of your own and after that gently bite it. Men like any time you steadily improve the pressure in that way, thus don't wait to nip him more demanding than you would love to be. Just in case you wanna be really extra, you're able to bring on an ice cube ahead of time for a lot more sensation.

## 15. The Dip Under his Ankle

Indeed, the location that usually gets fucked up if you are wearing brand new shoes! Involving your men's heel and s ankle there's a fingertip size stress point that can hold frustrating passion potential. This particular spot is attached to the sex organs and pressing it emits energy, producing thoughts of satisfaction.

Fix this: While in reverse cowgirl, grab the foot of his and also pulse every anxiety point of rhythm with the thrusts of your own. Do this right before he's intending to climax to really blow the head of his.

## 16. His Perineum

While he's afraid in the novice about living under the family jewels of his, the perineum is well worth the journey. This specific area of skin is situated in between the toes of his along with the anus of his plus it's right above his prostate gland - an organ with primary orgasmic power. A variety of mild strokes here can get him on the brink.

Fix this: Before he enters you in missionary, an entry in between the grab of his as well as lower limbs the penis of his. Then, press the knuckles of your own carefully into this particular area & start massaging. Right as he's planning to orgasm, press the knuckles of your own a little deeper to extend the fireworks.

## 17. His Shaft

The men sex organ...where to start? It's there. Everyone knows this is a huge part of sex. While you can try to have mastered the conventional practices and blow job, effort to spice things up with nearly anything fully uncharted like a reverse finger work.

Fix this: Make two little rings across the penis of his with the thumb of your own and index finger (like you're doing the okay hand symbol), stacking them one added to the next in the middle of the shaft of his. Twist the rings in opposite directions shifting from the facility with the best in addition to the foundation of the shaft of his also. Cox calls this a torrid twist the conventional one-handed uppy downy practical. Do not forget to utilize lube though!

## 18. The Head of his Penis

As most likely probably the most susceptible component of the penis, the top part may be a fickle art to master. It is able to effortlessly be difficult to locate the appropriate level of anxiety so you send him soaring into ecstasy but without recoiling in sensory overload.

Fix this: Give him a lipstick blow job - aka that you brush you're closed but relaxed mouth against the roof of the penis of his, like you're using lipstick. Maintain the shaft of his with the toes of your own, nonetheless, not in a fist (avoid always keeping the penis of his such as a mic, but do target it combined with exactly the same oblivious confidence of an average stand up act). Vary the thoughts by opening the mouth of your own a bit and massaging the top of his between them.

## 19. The Seam of his Testicles

Do you comprehend the location where Gepetto glued your boy's toes upon the body of his? And even love the way socks ordinarily have a seam in them? Successfully, your men' s got a digital camera that separates the testicles of his as well as will help them to remain from receiving one enormous test lump. It's a nerve abundant pleasure trail that runs top to bottom around the scrotum of his, as well as it's hugely underappreciated.

Fix this: Cradle the toes of his in one hand while thoroughly pressing the original two fingertips of the opposite hand of your own into the top of the crease (close to where testicles link on the basis of the penis) of his. Future trace downward with the toes of your own unless you reach the bottom part of the scrotum of his. But don't forget to be cautious!

## 20. His Frenulum

The F spot is the little nubbin of flesh below the crown of the penis of his linking the top of the shaft. it's normally lost since It's an element of the undercarriage, but there's truly a bundle of nerves just at that time that when touched tripped an amazing chain reaction of rapture.

Fix this: The the next time you're going down on him, maintain the penis of the constant of his thanks to one hand while really giving the crown of his your most. Each time you circle the tongue of your own around to the frenulum of his, flick it a few times along with your tongue stiffened, after which loosen up and also return to licking the crown.

## 21. His Lower Back

When you're looking for a way to transition the partner way TF of your own installed without truly spending the pants of his off, look no further. The pudendal nerve that stimulates the facets of the groin could be found, in the bottom with the spinal cord.

Fix this: Have your partner take the shirt of his off and lay on the belly of his with the arms of his by the edge of his. Hot tip: Keep the jeans of his on, but drive them down a couple of inches for a tantalizing hardly ever nude understanding. Lightly place the toes of your own or perhaps anxiety ravaged cuticles down throughout his lower back, stopping before you hit ass cheek.

## 22. The Earlobes of his

TBH, this is completely an underrated susceptible pocket of skin you're probably neglecting during your standard hookups - picture about exactly how jumpy you get when someone whispers in the ear of your own!

Fix this: Overstreet suggests kissing the partner of your own throughout the shoulder of his, up the neck of his, along with preventing before you reach the ear of his. Do this to each side, since asymmetry is created for any idle. When he's right about to lose it, start kissing the earlobe of his, and likewise use the tongue of your own to draw the earlobe of his into the jaws of your own. Play around with gentle nibbles, tongue, etc. Take care to not touch various other elements of the entire body of his while executing this particular, as well as to detect precisely how countryside he gets from you just touching the earlobes of his.

## THE WOMEN ORGASM

Orgasm is not just about pleasure. It is the same as an important requirement of women's overall health as it triggers the release of the stress hormones, which truly help the body unwind, minimize mental stress, help fight depression, and offer opportunities for full real physical and mental advancement. Find out all that you have to find out about this particular crucial feature of the body of your own under!

## What sorts of women orgasm are you going to recognize?

You are going to find three main types of women orgasm: clitoral, vaginal, and blended.

The clitoral orgasm is considered common. 70 5 % of women demand clitoral stimulation to attain orgasm. Vaginal orgasm means that women can achieve orgasm without any clitoral stimulation. Often this is through vaginal penetration. The most recent research, nevertheless, suggests that vaginal orgasm is just a misconception since the vagina is anatomically incapable of making an orgasm.

Ladies describe most likely the most enjoyable experiences to entail a mix of vaginal and clitoral orgasm. Furthermore in the list is definitely the many varieties: if the women encounter several orgasms in a row within a short time.

It seems like the prior two kinds are unusual, and only a couple of are in a place to experience.

G-Spot in women: where is it?
The G spot was present in 1950 by German gynecologist Ernst Greenberg, though the presence of its nevertheless comes about reasons.

Quite a few individuals believe it's an extension of the clitoris. Others believe the hype around this subject is useful simply to the producers of sex toys.

It's believed the G spot is situated on the front wall 0.8-1.2 in (2-3 cm) from the vagina entry. By touch, it's an estimated button and pressing on it may create a comprehensive bladder sensation. But after a while now, this particular feeling will vanish.

In a low number of jobs, the G spot stimulation can supply you with extraordinary sensations. Roughly 30 % of women suggest that vaginal orgasm in addition to pelvic muscle mass contractions are attained by the stimulation of the G spot during sex.

## What might result in an inability to orgasm?

According to a study, approximately thirty-three percent of women have not experienced an orgasm. The options of anorgasmia are split into two groups.

Psychological:
- irregular command over emotions, failing to disconnect
- poor self-esteem, fear of carrying out one thing wrong
- fear of getting pregnant
- damaging initial sexual experience
- psychological trauma
- stress

Physiological:

- hormonal disorders
- malfunctioning of the nervous and cardiovascular systems taking medications (especially antidepressants)

Most of the time, anorgasmia treatment is pushed by the real cause of the problem. Sometimes, it is adequate to check a fresh position or perhaps focus much more on foreplay to a climax. To read articles about furthermore, it can help, isn't it?

The lack of orgasm is seen normal at the beginning of one's sex life, when women's sexuality is awakening. In other cases, it might be a women orgasmic disorder plus an event to speak to a doctor.

Side effects of antidepressants: precisely how do they really influence libido and orgasms?
Almost all medications have negative effects, together with antidepressants aren't any different. Taking antidepressants might result in fat gain, nausea, or dizziness, though a strong matter is a minimal libido. Why does this happen?

Antidepressants work in the following way: they boost the quantity of serotonin, therefore bringing a sensation of calm and relaxation. At precisely the exact same time, it truly blocking the hormones responsible for arousal and prevents them from influencing specific structures of the human mind.

Decreased libido boasts a reduced production of good lubrication and postponed and even blocked orgasm.

Undoubtedly, every person responds in an alternative approach to antidepressants' sexual excess consequences, and the seriousness of them varies from situation to situation. Since antidepressants basically always provoke sexual problems, do not be embarrassed if you believe as you have been influenced by it. Discuss with the partner of your own as well as the physician of your own to establish the correct course of action.

**Non-vaginal orgasm: myth or fact?**

To stimulate the sex organs is considered typical, though not the single way to reach an orgasm. A few adult women orgasm, as an example, by the nipples of theirs getting rubbed. It has been established that in this specific scenario, the identical top area is aroused. One might come across orgasm while sleeping, obtaining one' s hair cut, performing exercising, hearing music, viewing racy films, or maybe just by the sturdiness of thought!

Nevertheless, it has to be noted that such techniques are usually much more of an exception instead of a rule. Don't read extraordinary into this specific. Only a bit of a proportion of women is able to buy it done, along with this is based on the mental state and biological attributes of the women.

**Many orgasms: could it be real?**
Many orgasms usually mean that getting numerous orgasms during one intercourse. For many women, multiple orgasms are attainable but just some are competent to

utilize the capability. Getting there requires effort and practice.

To begin, you would like a psychological setup. It is crucial being attuned to the idea that such pleasure is often obtained for you. You furthermore need to learn to listen to the body of your own and examine the erogenous zones you have.

Constant arousal is among the primary key problems for achieving correct multiple orgasms. Below, a terrific buy is determined by the partner. The partner of your own should keep on caressing you immediately after the very first orgasm of your own.

Often after orgasm, both the vagina and the penis become sensitive and further touch becomes unpleasant. In this specific scenario, one could promote various erogenous zones (the clitoris, the G-spot, the chest, the neck, etc.). To attain numerous orgasms, the understanding of the vagina is essential. You're able to enhance it by undertaking Kegel exercises teaching the vaginal muscles.

Orgasms along with age range Based on research, a woman is going to experience her most severe orgasm by the time she's 30 5. It is thought that at this particular age, she is satisfactory self-knowledge, confidence, together with sexual knowledge. That is everything necessary for top pleasure during sex.

That's the explanation thirty-year-old women have much more frequent & vivid orgasms compared with small people. Nevertheless, sensations do not end there. The study suggests that combined with the age gap, the sexual life of women becomes less arduous but much more sensual.

Contrary to stereotypes, the most effective orgasms can be found after menopause. This is associated with the drive to reside for one' s person, without any fear or maybe inhibition of unwanted pregnancy.

Just how Women Achieve Orgasm One of the ways women are in a position to really feel orgasm is by means of a goal-oriented 4 phase strategy at first talked about by the sex researchers William Masters and Virginia Johnson a lot of years ago.

1. Excitement In this specific state of desire or arousal, the woman initiates as well as agrees to sex, to ensure that since it commences she finds herself concentrating largely on sexual stimuli. Blood begins to engorge the clitoris, vagina, and nipples, and also produces a complete body sexual blush. Heart rate in addition to blood pressure levels increases. Testosterone in addition to neurotransmitters like dopamine and also serotonin are interested in these methods, says Dr. Ingber.

2. Plateau Sexual tension builds as a precursor to orgasm. The outside one-third of the vagina receives particularly engorged with blood, creating what researchers refer to as the "orgasmic platform." Focus on sexual stimuli drowns out other sensations. Pulse rate, blood pressure, and respiration continue and rise.

3. Orgasm Many rhythmic contractions occur in the uterus, vagina, and pelvic floor muscles. The sexual tension caused by lovemaking or maybe person stimulation releases, and groups of muscles with the body may contract. A feeling of warmth typically emanates from the pelvis as well as spreads through the entire body.

4. Resolution The body relaxes, with blood streaming separate from the engorged sexual organs. Pulse rate, blood pressure, and respiration go-to standard.

## MIND-BLOWING SEX POSITIONS FOR WOMEN

### 1. Corkscrew

Do It: Near the benefit of any bed or perhaps bench, sleeping on the hip in addition to forearm of one side and press the thighs of your own together. The partner stands of your own as well as straddles you, entering from behind.

Why: Keeping the thighs and legs of your own pressed collectively through this sex position offers for a tighter hold on him as he thrusts.

Enable it being Hotter: Instead of enabling the partner of your own do the efforts, try thrusting the hips of your own somewhat to enhance the tempo.

## 2. Face-Off

Do It: The partner of your own rests on a chair or the edge of the bed; you confront him, seated on the lap of his.

Why: During this specific sex position, you're in control of the perspective in addition to the level of the entry in addition to thrust. To be seated supplies help, consequently it's good for marathon sex sessions.

Enable it being Hotter: Let the toes of your own (and hands) do the talking. When seated, you're competent to put the hands of your own someplace on the body of your own or perhaps your partner's making things far more intriguing.

## 3. Doggy Style

Do It: Get on all fours, then possess the partner kneel of your own behind you, with his upper body straight up or perhaps rather draped over you (ya know, like a humping dog).

Why: This sex position allows effective penetration and less difficult G area stimulation.

Enable it being Hotter: Stimulate the clitoris of your own with one hand, and consult the partner of your own to do the finger process for you.

## 4. Pretzel Dip

Do It: Lie on your right side; your partner kneels, straddling the proper leg of your own and curling the left leg of your own close to the left aspect of his.

Why: With this specific sex position, you locate the considerably more extreme penetration of doggy look while constantly being able to produce that essential eye contact.

Enable it being Hotter: Get the partner of your own to massage the clit you have. Because, duh.

## 5. Flatiron

Do It: Lie facedown on the bed, legs and thighs straight, hips slightly raised.

Why: This sex position creates a snug fit, consequently your partner's penis will appear much larger.

Enable it being Hotter: Some shallow thrusts and deep breathing is able to assist the romp last longer.

## 6. G-Whiz

Do It: Lie once again in your lower limbs sitting on your partner's shoulders.

Why: This sex position is amazing as in case you boost the thighs and legs of your own, it narrows the vagina as well as let's concentrate on the G spot of your own.

Enable it being Hotter: Ask the partner of your own to start rocking you in a side-to-side or up-and-down motion. That can supply the penis into immediate exposure to the G spot of your own.

## 7. Cowgirl's Helper

Do It: The same as the preferred Cowgirl sex position, you kneel on top, pushing off your partner's chest and sliding up and down the thighs. Although the partner of your own aids by supporting a number of the weight of your own and getting your hips or thighs while he rises to meet up with each thrust.

Why: This sex position puts much less anxiety on the thighs and legs of your own, which helps make climaxing easier. Additionally, if you're with a fellow, women dominating sex positions postpone the climax of his - so everyone wins.

Allow it being Hotter: Alternate between shallow and deep thrusting to activate different areas of the vagina.

## 8. Wheelbarrow

Do It: Get on your hands and feet and in addition have him pick you instead by the pelvis. After gripping the waist of his with your thighs.

Why: Aside from being an excellent arm physical exercise for you, this men's dominant sex position allows him better penetration.

Enable it being Hotter: Try flooring a table or the side of the bed and provide the arms of your own a pause.

## 9. Leap Frog

Do It: This is an altered doggy style. Experiment with getting on your hands and knees, then, keeping hips raised, rest your head and arms on the base.

Why: This sex position creates increased penetration - and in addition provides a chance to rest on a pillow.

Enable it being Hotter: Make use of the hands of your own to advertise the clitoris of your own.

## 10. Remain and Deliver

Do It: With each people standing, you bend over in the waist; he enters you from behind.

Why: Bending over through this sex position is likely to create the vaginal walls tighter and improves the intensity of the friction.

Enable it being Hotter: Have your partner tickle the clitoris of your own with an entirely freehand, or possibly loosely connect the hands of your own combined with a silky scarf.

## 11. Secret Mountain

Do It: your partner sits, thighs & lower limbs bent, leaning back once again on his hands and forearms. You have to perform the actual same and after that inch toward him unless you're making contact.

Why: You'll both feel truly connected concentrating on each other. Increase the stimulation of your own by grinding the clitoris of your own contrary to the pelvis of his.

Enable it being Hotter: Slide ice cubes down the chest area of his and enable the great water gather on the basis of the pelvis of his.

## 12. Cowgirl

Do It: You kneel on top, pushing off your partner's chest and sliding up and down the thighs of his. You're competent to alleviate a number of the weight of your own from the pelvis of his by leaning back and also supporting yourself on the thighs of his.

Why: If it's the dominating in this sex position, you are going to postpone the climax of his as well as intensify yours.

Enable it being Hotter: Discover completely new sensations for equally people by widening the knee of your own or perhaps bringing them nearer to the entire body of his.

## 13. Overturn Cowgirl

Do It: The partner of your own is on the rear of his; you straddle him, dealing with the foot of his.

Why: This place enables you to take control and also clearly show the men of your own speed in addition to the rhythm you want.

Enable it being Hotter: To be able to have much more use, place your knees and shins within the thighs and legs of his and placed under the thighs of his.

## 14. Cowboy

Do It: You lie on the rear of your own even though the partner of your own straddles you. He next lightly inserts the penis of his through the little opening developed by the semi-closed legs you have.

Why: Tightness elevates the intensity of the penetration.

Enable it being Hotter: Have him fondle the breasts of your own and even gently hold on the wrists of your own for some bondage action.

## 15. Ballerina Dancer

Do It: Standing on one foot, deal with your partner and wrap another leg of your own all around the waist of his while he'll help support you.

Why: This sex position allows quality face time and also joining.

Enable it being Hotter: If you're genuinely flexible, think about putting the heightened leg on the shoulder of his for greater penetration.

## 16. Missionary

Do It: Do I just need to spell the pedometer out there? Okay. Lie on your rear while he's facedown along with you.

Why: This sex position is simple, elegant, effective, and surprisingly flexible. Vanilla, sure, but yummy.

Allow it being Hotter: You're competent to considerably modify the feeling for both people by changing the viewpoint of the thighs and legs of your own.

## 17. Cross-Booty

Do It: The partner of your own enters you from the missionary position, consequently slides his chest and legs out of the body of your own and so the pelvis of his is in the very same location but the limbs of his produce an X with yours.

Why: You are feeling a lot more of the entire body of his inactivity with this specific sex position.

Enable it being Hotter: Use this special perspective to massage the rear of his, butt, minimizing limbs as he thrusts. He is going to go nuts (as will you, watching him).

## 18. The Caboose

Do It: While he sits on the bed or a chair, back yourself in on the lap of his and scoop each other while seated.

Why: You can't find the partner of your own through this sex position, what this means is fantasizing is easier and can add to the excitement.
Enable it being Hotter: Tighten the muscles of the pelvic floor of your own so you're competent to keep him & keep him hard AF.

## 19. Scoop Me Up

Do It: Both of you lie on your sides, facing precisely exactly the same track. You bring the knee of your own up somewhat while the partner of your own slides up turning the pelvis of your own as well as enters you from behind. (You may additionally understand this as spooning.)

Why: This sex position allows for far more skin-to-skin contact, improving the stimulation of your own.

Enable it being Hotter: Have your partner place the hands of his on the shoulders of your own to increase the intensity in addition to the deepness of the thrust.

## 20. Overturn Scoop

Do It: From the missionary position, without disengaging, switch in concert upon the sides of your own, making use of the arms of your own to permit top of the bodies of your own.

Why: You get precisely the same complete body press and can gaze into each other' s eyes.

Enable it being Hotter: Try intertwining the thighs and legs of your own with his or maybe fondling him down under.

## 21. Golden Arch

Do It: your partner rests with the thighs and legs of his straight as well as you stay additionally to him with knees which are bent beside the thighs of his, as well as you both lean back.

Why: This location gives you both great views of each other's s bodies which are complete. You'll similarly have command with the depth, speed, and perspective of the thrusts.

Enable it being Hotter: Have him work together with the hands of his to massage the clitoris of your own, and have your own. Lean back farther for additional G area stimulation.

## 22. The Seashell

Do It: Lie once again in your legs raised the way up and your ankles crossed behind the unique head of your own. He enters you beginning out of a missionary position.

Why: The hands of your own are free to do the clitoris of your own. As you have to.

Enable it being Hotter: Have him use incredibly high, massaging the pubic bone of his against the clitoris of your own, and perhaps drive low, solely revitalizing the G spot of your own combined with the roof of the penis of his.

## 23. Butter Churner

Do It: Lie on your rear jointly with the lower limbs of your own elevated and folded over therefore the lower legs of your own are on every aspect of the top of your own, while he squats and dips the penis of his in and from the vagina of your own.
Why: Aside from getting that eye contact, the extra dash of blood at the top of your own will boost the ecstasy.

Enable it being Hotter: Have him dribble dairy chocolate syrup or perhaps something sweet in the mouth of your own (yes, really). It gets a lot more of your senses needed, amping up the entire experience.

## 24. The Chairman

Do It: your partner rests on the edge of the foundation as well as you keep on him, facing away.

Why: This sex position will reach the spots in, the G spot of your own. Meanwhile, you're competent to utilize the hands of your own to promote his scrotum or perineum.

Enable it being Hotter: Bring the knee of your own closer to the chest of your own, supporting the foot of your own on the base.

## 25. The Pinball Wizard

Do It: You have a partial bridge work (like a pinball machine), along with your weight flooring the shoulders of your own. The partner of your own enters you from a kneeling position.

Why: It provides for the partner of your own fast entry to trigger the clitoris of your own and also massage the mons pubis.

Enable it being Hotter: Throw one leg up against the shoulder of his for deeper penetration.


## 26. Valedictorian

Do It: From a missionary position, you boost your thighs and legs and grow them directly through (forming a V).

Why: This allows body contact which is good with all of the vulva.

Allow it being Hotter: Try obtaining your lower legs. It's in a position to supply you with stability as well as an additional stretch to boost the sensation.

## 27. Spork

Do It: As you lie on the rear of your own, boost the proper leg of your own so he's in a position to put himself between the thighs and legs of your own in a ninety-degree angle and enter you. The thighs and legs of your own will develop the tines of a spork (that's a scoop fork combo, ICYDK). You're competent to achieve this with him facing you or maybe confronted with the rear of your own. Options!

Why: From the spork work, you're competent to increase the best leg of your own and also aid it by sleeping it on your partner's shoulder. From here, you're able to easily stimulate your clitoris with the toes of your own while he is within you.

Allow it being Hotter: Synchronize the breath you have. One people take the lead along with the various other uses so you consume & exhale together. The coordinated rhythm opens an unspoken dialogue of intimacy.

## 28. Seated Wheelbarrow

Do It: Have your partner stay in the advantage of any bed or perhaps a chair and position yourself therefore the butt of your own is in the lap of his, and expand the hands of your own securely on the floor. Extend the legs of your own out behind the waist of his (it'll probably work well if he supports the thighs) of your own plus pump away.

Why: This position allows strong penetration - and also you are going to work the arms of your own while you're at it.

Enable it being Hotter: Try rhythmically squeezing the pelvic muscle tissues of your own, to help you each attain a strong climax.

## 29. Dinner table Top

Do It: You don't have to do this one on a table - each surface region that hits the partner of your own at crotch level will do. Have him enter you while you're resting or even possibly sleeping in the advantage of a table, counter, and maybe even the bed of your own.

Why: This location is great for face-to-face action. Furthermore, just in case you two are relatively various heights, this is an excellent option, since it places you both at the identical height.

Enable it being Hotter: Try getting the thighs and legs of your own down and putting the foot of your own on the chest area of his, prior to the shoulders of his. This allows you to deal with the tempo in addition to the depth of thrusts.

## 30. Champagne Room

Do It: Your partner sits as well as you stay additionally to him, facing away.

Why: It is able to enable you to manage the speed in addition to the intensity of the thrusts.

Allow it being Hotter: Try doing it on the stairs or the edge of the tub. Involves a bit of talent...but hey, practice makes perfect, amirite?

## 31. The Om

Do It: The partner of your own sits cross-legged (yoga/pretzel style), you stay in his lap facing him. Wrap the thighs and legs of your own about him and hug each other for support.

Why: Best for tantric sex. Rocking, not thrusting, will be the crucial component with respect to its truly personal spot.

Enable it being Hotter: Lock to each other' s deep gaze to put extra oh in on the big O.

## 32. Upstanding Citizen

Do It: You straddle him, wrapping the thighs and your legs close to the entire body of his (he is going to keep his hips unlocked and thighs spread slightly). He appears as well as supports you in the arms of his. You're competent to start on the foundation and in addition have him pick you in position without any disengaging. (Or just for the genuinely daring, you're in a position to hop aboard from standing position!)

Why: This is the positioning of every steamy romance movie...a.k.a, it's a must-try.

Enable it being Hotter: Have him drive you up against a framework - rather carefully.

## 33. The Spider

Do It: Sit on the bed with legs toward one another, arms to guide yourselves. Today move collectively & upon the penis of his. The hips of your own are gonna be in between the spread legs of his, the knee of your own bent, and feet outside of the hips of his and dull on the base. Now rock back and forth.

Why: You're competent to actually keep eye contact while checking out the action at the center stage.

Enable it being Hotter: Grab your partner's hands and pull yourself in place inside a squatting position while he's returned. Or perhaps he's in a position to remain seated upright and help you move contrary to the chest of his in on the Lazy Man work.

## 34. The Good Ex

Do It: Sit on the bed facing each other with legs forward. Increase your partner's best leg with the left of your own and raise the proper leg of your own with the left of his. Come together so he's in a position to jump into you. Nowadays both of you lie once again, your legs building an X. Slow, simple gyrations shift thrusting.

Why: Prolonged easy sex and that will construct the arousal of your own. Shallow thrusts stimulate the nerve endings in the roof of the penis of his.

Enable it being Hotter: Reach out and hold hands to pull together for pelvic thrusting. Furthermore, alternate alternatively sitting up and he lies once again without changing the rhythm.

## 35. The Lazy Man

Do It: Place pillows driving your partner's back and in addition have him remain on the bed with legs outstretched. Now straddle the waist of his, legs on the base. Bend the knee of your own to lower yourself onto him, making use of one hand to level the penis of his in. By simply pressing on the toes of the foot of your own and releasing, you're competent to raise and lower yourself upon the shaft of his as steadily and even as quickly as you do.

Why: This location puts you in command, plus maintains a great deal of intimacy. Consider the penis of his as a masturbatory tool, one thing to massage and also trigger the clitoris of your own with and against.

Enable it being Hotter: From this particular school, you both might lie back once again into the Spider job or perhaps its a lot more challenging variation, the Good Ex.

## 36. Ice Angel

Do It: Lie on your rear as well as have your partner straddle you dealing with away. Lift up the legs of your own and wrap them all around the rear of his to raise the pelvis of your own so he's in a position to get into you. Get the butt of his to help him slide up and also returned. Include just a bit of massage action on the grip of your own.

Why: You are going to get a prime view of the adorable butt of his. In addition, due to this place, you have access which is very easy to fondle the testicles of his. To not note, the pelvis of his is adequately placed to grind against the clit of your own.

Enable it being Hotter: Have him spin around into missionary style to you've while trying to stay introduced. Then switch positions, this time together with you on top & face at bay.

## 37. Wrapped Lotus

Do It: Have your partner sit cross-legged along with climb in the lap of his, facing him, together with the lower limbs of your own wrapped all around the rear of his. Have your partner enter you and grind up against the pelvis of his.

Why: This position allows for many primary face-to-face intimacy. In addition there's a lot of room for creativity in this specific spot - which includes revitalizing different erogenous zones on each others' good bodies, the same as the head, neck, and expertise.

Enable it being Hotter: Ask him to lick the nipples of your own and allow his hands roam. Plus roam...and roam. (You get the idea.)

## 38. The Snake

Do It: Lie down on the belly of your own, as well as have your partner lie down along with you and slide in from behind.

Why: This position allows for very rich penetration, together with a snug fit which will truly look amazing for you along with the partner of your own.

Enable it being Hotter: You're competent to reach again and also wrap the hand of your own all around the shaft of his to enable you to manage precisely how deeply he becomes or even switch up the viewpoint of the butt of your own because of the identical outcome.

## 39. Woman Astride

Do It: This location is just like a cowgirl, but with a twist. Climb on top as well as have your partner enter you. Then, lean back and place the hands of your own on the bed for help, building a forty-five-degree angle on your partner's legs.

Why: This alteration of perspective aids concentrate on the G spot of your own much more, and additionally gives you command with speed in addition to the number of thrusts. Furthermore, the partner of your own has an entry which is very easy on the clitoris of your own.

Enable it being Hotter: Give yourself a hand with the "V stroke": Make a V with the list in addition to the ring finger of a single hand and place the toes on each aspect of the clitoris of your own with the penis of his in between. Drive the toes of your own down in a rocking motion.

## 40. Abdominal Down

Do It: Lie on the belly of your own with the hand's thrust of your own between the thighs and legs of your own. Grind the thighs and legs of your own also and together shift the hips of your own down plus up consequently the clitoris of your own and also pubic mound rub against your properly held fingers.

Why: Simple but superb satisfaction.

Allow it being Hotter: It's easy to add to most back entry positions, like the Flatiron or perhaps the Leapfrog.

## 41. Bubble the Fun

Do It: Having the body submerged minimizing limbs dangling out of the tub, start through yourself a rubdown up best before you are able to go right down to roam around under the water.

Why: Relaxing in a comfy, nice smelling foot bath can help relieve stress, ease stress, as well as definitely gets you in the mood.

Enable it being Hotter: Include a waterproof vibe creating waves or perhaps use your respective removable shower head (may I recommend the "pulse" setting?). Steady streams of h2o on the clitoris can be quite pleasant.

## 42. Hunt and also Learn

Do It: Holding a hand mirror, stay in a comfy seat with one leg propped up on the base as well as a couch. Because you're competent to check out the merchandise, venture far out of your weak clitoris to discover out new erogenous zones. Check out the opening, inside, and back wall system of the vagina of your own jointly in your fingers, pressing, and changing strain until you find out something that looks perfect Positive Many Meanings - - Positive Many Meanings.

Why: It may look elementary, although you get a novice driver's point of view. You may discover a fresh strategy to "ring your bell," that will help relieve the frustration numerous women think when they're able to are made in only one position.

Enable it being Hotter: Check it out together with the favored sex toy of your own, or perhaps possess the partner slide of your own in from the Seashell or perhaps possibly Butter Churner work.

## 43. Team Perk

Do It: From a seated position, do the finger of your own to get a group within the clitoris of your own. Start slowly and boost speed and pressure, based on the response of your own.

Why: This move is great for women which find immediate clitoral strain far too intense for lengthy stimulation.

Allow it being Hotter: Fed up together with the O shape? Test with tracing the letters of the alphabet on the clit of your own to vary the sensation.

## 44. Couch Grind

Do It: Ride the arm of a stuffed chair or couch, or maybe perhaps the benefit of any table or perhaps a table with a huge towel or blanket folded over it. Start with a small motion of the hips, furthermore steadily create momentum.

Why: Great if you prefer sound, constant strain on the clitoris of your own.

Allow it being Hotter: Feeling a little overly American Pie? Grip the arm with the thighs of your own as well as have the man of your own end up in you from behind. Easily make sure never to break some furniture.

## 45. Try getting on the G-Spot

Do It: Lie on the rear of your own and bring the knee of your own in towards the chest of your own. Insert one or perhaps two toes heavily into the vagina of your own. As you withdraw the finger of your own, media against the front aspect of your vagina and urethra and curl the finger of your own in a beckoning gesture.

Why: On this particular movement, it's typical to feel little urgency to urinate in the novice, however with many practice and sessions, you're able to appear to feel a brilliant, experience that is enjoyable.

Enable it being Hotter: Try it with only 1 leg bent on the chest of your own, extending the other, for a variation on the sense.

## 46. Faucet Dance

Do It: Lie on one side with one leg extended and definitely the complete opposite bent. With a single hand, carefully distinct & store the labia of your own on the sides, and additionally apply a little drop of lube in your exposed clitoris. Next, with the opposite hand, begin tapping correctly on it.

Why: Tapping, instead of rubbing, might lead to quick and intense sensations for people who find immediate stimulation excessively arduous.

Allow it being Hotter: Tapping more quickly or even harder can establish unique sensations. Determine just how long you're competent to keep going or even consult the partner of your own to participate in the fun.

## THE PENIS SIZE WOMEN PREFER

News which is great, typically endowed men of the planet! In terms of penis size, bigger isn't frequently better! Although it doesn't damage being slightly above average...

According to the researchers:

"Women preferred a penis of relatively larger length as well as circumference for one period (length = 6.4 inches/16.3 cm, circumference = 5.0 inches/12.7 cm) as compared to long-range (length = 6.3 inches/16.0 cm, circumference = 4.8 inches/12.2 cm) sexual partners."

Almost all those values are relatively larger as opposed to the typical American penis size: approximately 5.6 inches in length also as 4.8 inches in circumference when totally erect.

The researchers observed that women might not like a lot larger penises on account of their possible to tear or even damage the really vulnerable buildings inside the vagina.

"Anything which raises friction during intercourse might promote genital damage, indirectly boosting infection danger. A larger phallus would boost friction loved one to a lessened phallus. These potential issues associated with a larger penis suggest precisely why the men penis has not created to be larger," the researchers noted

Some other interesting tidbits from the study: 20 7 % of the subjects found they would end a relationship partly due to a mismatch in the ideal penis size of theirs together with their partner's genitalia. Nevertheless, 80 3 % of the respondents stated they'd been present as centered on penis size as various women or maybe not concerned about it at all.

An important power of the evaluation was the usage of its three-dimensional guide objects in addition to a study appear where subjects actually answered questions in the lab. Nevertheless, these methodological strengths restricted the size in addition to the range of the participant group. Subjects tended to be younger and were recruited on the UCLA campus. You won't ever know whether the preferences of theirs are going to match those of women throughout the nation?

A prior analysis demonstrated that around 2 thirds of men agonize inevitably regarding the size of the part of theirs, along with a lot of truly consider methods to better the sizes of the phallus of theirs.

But rather than popping penis enlargement pills which don't do the job, men will likely be far better to do not stressing about the genitalia of theirs, being cozy in who they are, and finding out how to utilize the complete repertoire of materials in the disposal of theirs for sexual pleasure.

## THINGS WOMEN DO THE MEN FIND IRRESISTIBLE

While heels and a small dress might catch the eye of his, it is not always the type of stuff that actually hooks him in. Truth be told, men are focusing on the small stuff also. he is noticing her tuning and quirks in on the nervous tics of her because at the conclusion of the day, it is the small stuff He is falling for and is not in a position to resist. Men are not as oblivious as we believe, and we should really provide them with much more credit for focusing on the manner in which we tie the hair of ours or maybe the reality that we could install a television on our own. What we may believe is "normal" may just be the point that catches the eye of his and perhaps even the heart of his.

## Women Without Any Makeup

Unbelievably, though many men like the ladies of theirs being au naturel. You may be pleasantly surprised to find out that women might invest near to 1dolar1 200,000 on skincare products in a lifetime. That is outrageous. Though it is since we have a concept that we have to conceal ourselves from men. "When a woman does not wear make-up, the natural beauty of her is on display. Additionally, some men think it is a massive turn-off to kiss women and discover that they're smeared with lipstick. Make-up can occasionally act like a barrier instead of a come-on."

## Girls With Smudged Makeup

You may find this one a bit weird, but it is real. Much love bedhead allures men, smudged cosmetics does exactly the same thing. It provides you with that tussled, just-rolled-out-of-bed appearance as well as men are around which. Women typically get that look whenever they forget to draw the makeup of theirs off at night. "Men get this [attractive] since you look as you have only produced love. It reminds them of just how good the afterglow [is]." It is not surprising that men find it irresistible.

## Sense Of Smell

You may be imagining there is no chance a fellow understands when a woman is ovulating, but naturally, they actually do. Men can literally smell a woman who is ovulating without truly knowing it. Men know when a woman is prepared and can find them a lot more appealing during this time. Of the research, it was discovered that men's testosterone measurements spiked whenever they smelled a women's garments which she was wearing when she was ovulating. It surely goes to a men's natural instinct to procreate.

## Texting Him If You Get Home

Girls who text the boyfriend of theirs after they've had several are more appealing to men. You most likely assumed your men found it annoying whenever you will blow up the phone of his right after a night out together with the women, but that is not the situation in all. Men like it when we copy them since it will make them feel needed, particularly since they're most likely currently thinking whether you're obtaining hit on. "Letting folks understand how you think is equally reassuring & appealing. All of us love compliments."

## Girls Wearing Ball Caps

Regardless of whether you're planning to view a live baseball game or simply creating a casual working day, men can't get plenty of seeing their girlfriends sporting ball caps, and more particularly, seeing a ponytail with a ball cap. There is simply a thing about it men discover really foxy. Sometimes, it actually does not take up very much to impress men and it is generally when you're at your most casual he finds you probably the foxiest.

## Stretching It Out

In case you have already seen that while you're in the gym stretching, you have a tendency to capture a men 's eye, it is simply because men discover women that stretch to be desirable. We may think it is to be strange, but men find it irresistible. Those average involuntary motions that you are making while you're stretching are in fact irresistible to men. Amusing enough, among the largest on the list may be the stretch in which the arms of your own are high up in the atmosphere. You can bet the men that go to the yoga classes of your own are watching out the entire time.

**Not Planning**

Men adore it if you do not consider it very difficult and in most cases, whenever they see a woman with coordinating undergarments, they assumed you'd much more designed for the evening. Women who are found with mismatched undergarments possibly came unprepared or simply did not care about such things. "Men like getting you in mismatching [undergarments] since appears as you were not thinking about anything at all, though they have managed to persuade you." Just another small peek into a men's brain.

## Giving Up On The Heels

Whether or not you are simply chilling at home, relaxing in the park, or even hitting up the dance flooring with bare legs, there is simply a thing about women ditching the shoes of her which manages to do it for men. She simply looks as she is in her comfortable and natural state. "Bare foot has got a hint of nudity. Walking barefoot implies naturalness along with a rebel against convention, and may clue a man into fantasies of wildness."

## Perfect The Hair Flip

One more subconscious movement you make that men find irresistible is if you flip the hair of your own. Men seriously cannot get enough of this basic movement. In case you remember in many romantic comedies, you are going to see this particular gesture since a lot of women understand it is something that will capture a men 's eye. When you are able to be a master to do the flip, you can easily rule the household of your own with only a flip of the hair of your own. It has one easy gesture which works wonders.

## When She will Goof Off With Him

A girl who's in a position to goof off around the men of her is extremely attractive because it shows you know the way to have a great time. Any kind of outside-the-box behavior will keep a man interested since it shows him you are not like some other girls. Not merely is it fun, though it shows you're a confident woman. An Australian study previously showed that non-conformists are viewed as a lot better than conformists. A woman who can fool around is one who does not care what others believe and it is ready to accept having fun with the man of her.

## Getting The Punch Line Wrong

Consider the final time you attempted to tell the man of your own a joke and also you completely messed it up? You most likely felt really foolish, but odds are, your men thought it had been pretty attractive. Men love silly girls since they're less intimidating.

"Men is usually intimidated by intellectual women, therefore acquiring it wrong makes her much less intimidating and they are able to unwind in the company of her. It shows the triggers and vulnerability of his protective instinct."
And so the next time you blunder a laugh, do not care about it.

**Girls Who Laugh Out Loud**

We have all been there when we're relaxing in a team of someone and people in the team burst out laughing with probably the most rambunctious laugh. A number of individuals discover a type of laughter annoying, but several men believe that it is great foxy.

## Making The First Move

You will be thinking, there's simply no chance you are making the very first move, but there are a variety of men that cannot get plenty of it. One study which dealt with speed dating discovered that connections might be built through women showing interest. This not merely is true for the very first date, but to the whole relationship. He is going to love it each time you make the very first action.

## Reading In Bed

A man discovers a woman that reads silently in bed to be extremely foxy. Perhaps it is the soft lighting or perhaps it is the reality that you look content while you're reading, no matter, men loving seeing their women read. It can possibly have a great deal to do with the reality that it is an unbiased act. It is not a process that you simply need him to become a part of. A number of couples love to read together or even have one partner read on the other person. Anything you men love to do in concert, rest assured, the men of your own love this process of your own.

## Wearing His Clothes

Men go insane over this. There's simply something about a woman who wears her men's clothing which drives him wild. You have to to use the shirt in only the proper way which means oversized with the bare legs of your own. Do not forget to leave 3 buttons unbuttoned for maximum impact. Women typically realize that This is one thing that men find attractive, therefore you might have tried this technique out previously. It is a surefire method to get your men's interest.

## Touch

Actual physical contact is an enormous turn-on for men, when applied the proper way. It is an enormous turn-on for girls, also. Though these days we are talking about what men find irresistible.

As a fast digression, I simply wanted to mention I make use of the terms girls and women interchangeably. I ought to have pointed out this earlier. I was raised just south of Boston, so we call adult women, women. I recognized that various other areas of the nation do not do it when I was in the teens of mine, going close to the nation playing guitar in a band. Nevertheless, simply so you realize, when I say women I merely mean women.

Okay, again to touch. A properly positioned hand, operating the fingers of your own up the arm of ours, or having a hug only a bit more than expected can easily acquire men wild.

You won't believe that men notice these issues. Nevertheless, oh, the way we do!

**Glasses**

To wear glasses may totally alter the way someone looks. A pair of reading glasses are able to make women appear much more intellectual. A pair of huge, round sunglasses are able to make a women look relaxed & confident.

A lot of men as women that wear glasses. They are not simply for nerds anymore!

Men notice when a woman is wearing glasses. And we particularly notice when a woman that often wears glasses, is not wearing them.

There is a well used saying: Men do not make passes at women that use glasses. Now, I do not know if perhaps this used to be accurate if the saying originated. But it is certainly not true today.

A lot of men essentially prefer a woman that wears glasses. There is a wide variety of types currently available you are able to buy the perfect glasses to complement the personality of your own. Like clothing, the choice of your own in glasses is able to say a great deal about who you're.

If you are women and you're self-conscious about the glasses of your own (as some women are), do not be. There is a lot of men available that discover them attractive.

**Breath**

The final item on the list of ours of items that you won't think men find appealing about women is the breath of her.

Clearly, if a woman has bad breath, it is a turn-off. But you will find a few things about a women's breath that men find sexy.

For starters, if a woman gets near adequate to a fellow that he is able to really feel the breath of her, it is often a turn on. Leaning in and whispering a thing right into a men 's ear, regardless of what's said, can easily send a chill down a men's back.

The next thing about a women's breath which- Positive Many Meanings- men notice will be the speed. A woman that shoots very long, deep breaths comes across as being calm & confident. Rapidly, breathing that is shallow is going to make a woman come across as anxious and flighty.

You might not believe that men notice this, though we quite often do. And it is never on a conscious level. Body language, voice, posture, and breathing rate all communicate exactly how you are feeling inside.

## Women Irresistible Traits

### 1. Confidence

She does not have a huge ego, mind you. Though she feels secure in who she's as well as assumes she's incredible in the own right of her. She commands respect just by the way in which she carries herself. She understands the way to set boundaries and look after the emotional needs of her.

She shows that she's truly keen on learning what's additionally awesome about the man she's just met. Graphic being he's, small escapes the notice of his as he appreciates exactly how she carries herself, the dresses she is wearing, her hair, her walk, her all.

Confidence in women is extremely appealing and also really gorgeous.

## 2. Physical magnetism

What makes a woman irresistible and originally attracts men is body language through external appearances. She's nicely groomed as well as takes pride in each and every detail of the appearance of her, not just the dresses she's wearing or maybe the manner in which she wears her makeup and hair.

She looks both properly dressed and sexually appealing as well as has got the small things, like well-manicured nails, very good oral hygiene, a subtle and soft scent rather than reeking of perfume. Men discover all of the small details and value a woman that looks after the appearance of her from the inside out.

## 3. A tasteful sense of humor

A woman who smiles shows she's usually a lucky person. She's not shallow and doesn't laugh too frequently or even very long at what might not be funny enough. Nor does she agree too rapidly before he's expressed any actual ideas or points, sometimes.

And above all, she's never ever sarcastically amusing or even makes jokes at her date 's expense. She's sincere and skips the sharp-edged wit. An excellent sense of humor is a women's greatest advantage.

## 4. Full-on presence

She's focused on what a man is thinking rather than fidgeting with shuffling, her hair, or her napkin through some other views like, I think about what he does? or maybe How can I look? or perhaps Will he be the men I marry? The mind of her is completely crisp plus she hears the text of the men she's with rather than remaining psychologically distracted.

She appears at him while he is talking and it is actually devoted to listening. He is able to feel the attention of her, the eyes of her on the lips of his, and the reaction of her to the words he's saying. There's nothing much more romantic than letting the men she's with know she's entirely present with him.

## 5. Passion

She's enthusiastic about herself, the beliefs of her, what is essential to her on the planet. She's passionate when sharing the ideas of her, her family, her art, her job, her hobby, or maybe anything it's that she's into.

It does not matter what it's she is conveying. she is letting him determine what she desires in daily life and what She is actively pursuing. When he hears the passion of her, he's in a position to realize her better as well as realize that she is going to support whatever it's he could be interested in.

## 6. Intelligence

Women who could hold a respectful, decent, and smart discussion is admirable.

She demonstrates that she is able to keep her own in virtually any environment, at every conference, in a restaurant, or perhaps at any family event and gathering. She's a woman he's proud to present to his family and friends.

## 7. Independence

Men admire a woman with a fulfilling life, who's got plenty of friends, has activities which she really loves for getting involved in, whose job is extremely fulfilling to her, who's independent, and who don't rely on him for the happiness of her.

## 8. Appreciation

Any woman who shows the appreciation of her for those that the partner of her does wins the heart of his. Acknowledgment as well as appreciation are the gas a man uses in a relationship. Far more than anything, he really needs her in order to recognize as well as validate him and also to allow him to know he will make her happy by all he brings to the connection.

## 9. Value

Men love to know they are providing a thing of great value on the relationship, a feeling of purpose and mission. A woman who makes men feel needed as well as valued makes him would like to love and take care of her more deeply.

## 10. Loyalty

For men, love is commitment. They recognize a woman who is going to stand by them regardless of what happens. This consists of setbacks in life.

For instance, in case the business of his views a downturn also he can't carry home almost as he would once, or even in case the health of his suffers plus he wants her to stand by him and foster him. If the loyalty of her is unimpeachable and real, she is going to have him for life.

## 11. Calm demeanor

A proper, masculine man is turned off by women who are too talkative or perhaps who brags about herself as well as the accomplishments of her. He can't hold on to the masculinity of his in the presence of her and can often feel emasculated or even leave. He appreciates women and has a calm presence.

## 12. Knows how you can receive

She likes feeling cherished & pampered, to keep men opened the automobile door for her, get proper care of her, hold the hand of her when crossing the avenues, and also be conscious of her in public and also among family and friends. She feels nurtured and protected and safe, and the graciousness of her makes the men feel he's needed and valued.

He views through the actions of his which she is happy, and also since she appreciates and also recognizes him, he feels as he's received her over.

## 13. Believe in her personal opinion

He respects a woman that knows and trusts in what she desires and it is cozy in articulating the opinions of her and the needs of her. Forming views of him depending on what the friends of her or maybe family members believe, psychologically inviting individuals to sit down on the judges' board and maybe disqualify him right after they meet up with is a huge error.

It doesn't give her an opportunity to get to learn the actual individual he's. Numerous women have the practice of testing the men they meet all over their initial date instead of giving themselves permission to learn precisely what they might like about one another.

# SECURE METHODS TO INCREASE WOMEN LIBIDO

Every woman is able to experience reduced libido at some stage. Discover how to restore it along with a couple of recommendations below that might are available in handy for you.

Causes of low libido Decreased libido of women are able to occur at any time after you have become sexually active. Many women experience it a great deal after pregnancy when breastfeeding.

Additionally, the libido of your own may go crashing from 100 back to 0 because of anxiety, stress, or maybe hormonal imbalance because of changes within the body. Often a particular level of sexual disorder is able to cause loss of libido of women.

Whatever function as the reason behind your reduced libido, it should not cause you much more tension or even function as the main reason you shy from attempting to obtain- Positive Many Meanings - the green light on once again for the partner of your own. Precisely why is the fact that? Lowered libido is not a sentence and you'll find ways that are different to boost it.

## Ways To Increase Women Libido

Exercise much more Different household remedies and cures are present, several of that you are able to whip up by yourself to have your sexual drive up. Among the causes for lack of sex drive of women may be a shortage of physical exercise. Exercise is required for an optimally balanced body therefore the doctor of your own may recommend to add it to the list of your own of things that are healthy to help you boost the libido of your own.

Exercising much more than your everyday walk to the market or even to that park nearby is the very best natural libido booster you are able to get for free. It may simply set you back a couple of drops of sweat though but what's that when compared with the pleasure which will come with having the libido of your own back.

Investigate the libido of your own Whatever exercise you've to do; whether it is yoga or simply operating from a few blocks to the next or even running about the park, when it allows you to hook far more to the body of your own and also be conscious of your own self, you're a stride to skyrocketing that libido next. Nearly all physicians advise physical exercise because it will allow you to feel a great deal far more at ease and confident in the room.

You know one activity that provides you guts? Taking boxing class. You can try out that as you may have all of the guts as well as the confidence you are able to buy when you're running a case of decreased libido due to self-esteem that is low or maybe mental health problems.

Specific pelvic exercises may also go quite a distance to help your muscle mass relax so in case the doctor of your own indicates Kegels to help the pelvic region of your own as the muscles around generally there are accountable for contraction throughout orgasm, then follow the recommendations of her. You just don't know, it may be that missing piece you have not tried yet.

Cope with stress Learning to deal with stress in a good way is able to improve women's sex drive. Rubbing your anxiety and stress in the face of his does not help him recognize just how stressed you're, it just provides him much more tension more particularly when he's been attempting to help you aroused all to no avail. Eliminate the stress of your own somehow.

The doctor of your own might suggest meditation. That is one of the greatest methods to cope with the stress of your own. Anytime you're feeling your anxiety topping the charts, you are able to get into the room of your own or maybe anything else place which is quiet that you have chosen, clear the head of your own of all of the troubling ideas meditate on just how lovely life is as well as the reality that having the partner of your own yet craving for you personally is among the very best things ever. Look at stress as a call to action as respect the lifestyle of your own and make changes that are positive on yourself with it.

After you have dealt with all of the stress, the body of your own is going to relax and also you can have the libido of your own back and intact.

Talk to the partner of your own Spending time and also speaking with your partner goes a great deal of approach to help you also in the game. Every single woman, regardless of how busy you receive, ought to invest a minimum of twenty mins of talking time with the partner of her. This time must be only for the partner of your own and never interrupted by any electronics or social media.

Communication is able to help him understand just how to enable you to get the libido of your own back. It will aid him to recognize if prolonged foreplay is going to do the key for yourself or even possibly speaking in a sensuous method to you. Nevertheless it might be, put aside partner time and talk.

Enhance the love life of your own Having just one specific prim as well as correct method to initiate sex each time may cause women libido issues. Sex becomes boring and also you steadily lose interest. At this stage, spicing up the love life of your own by coming up with various additional methods to arouse your teaching or spouse him many other methods for getting you in the game may go a great deal of way to tackle your reduced libido.

**Get lots of sleep**

A busy lifestyle is able to snatch the precious sleep of your own from you and thus making weary and also stressed out. Sleep allows your nerves unwind and in turn will help the body of your own to function typically. If the body gets less sleep and much more stressed out, you have a tendency to lose interest in a number of issues. Exhaustion reduces the sex drive of your own therefore getting plenty of rest or even using power naps if you are able to while accompanying it with the rich-in-protein eating plan is able to go quite a distance in boosting your sex drive.

Sex drive foods Eating a great deal more chocolate could be which home cure that matches your needs. You know what they are saying about milk chocolate and also the reality that it symbolizes drive. This is not simply due to its mind-blowing taste which sets the taste buds of your own on longing and fire for more when it is available in contact with them.

A report done on chocolate shows it can help in the secretion of even more serotonin in the body of your own. Medical professionals around the globe point out this hormone is liable for placing you in an aphrodisiac mood. Guess what it really does to the body of your own? It longs for a men touch after a serving of chocolates or various other pleasurable food as figs, peaches or oysters. You could opt to combine the two popular aphrodisiacs: oysters and chocolate.

If consuming these 2 receives you feeling sensuous and feels enjoyable, then get prepared to be fired in place for a very long period of action. Dealing with yourself to a homemade recipe with these 2 as dessert could leave you wanting a much more than dessert to satisfy the sensuous perception it's awoken.

Consuming a great deal of fruit could be an additional good house therapy for a lowered sex drive of women. A few certain fruits have been discovered as well as recommended by physicians for consumption during this particular time of the life of your own as a woman. Aside from the fruits already stated, various other fruit like bananas, moreover avocado not merely boost the libido of your own but additionally increases blood circulation on the genitals and consequently advertising a healthy and normal sex life.

Make a scheduled appointment for your practitioner Consulting the health practitioner of your own for a case of reduced libido is among probably the wisest foods you need to do before you get started on any form of therapy or treatment.

Whether or maybe not you believe that the organic approach will be the very best for you, making a scheduled appointment for your medical practitioner to allow him or perhaps her know about the libido problems of your own are able to go quite a distance that will help you find out in case the libido issue of your own is simply due to anxiety or even some other fundamental issues. Most times the libido of your own might be as an outcome of women's lubrication problems or maybe various other underlying health conditions which may be mental or otherwise.

Regardless of the issue may be, the doctor of your own is going to be the only person to allow you to realize the root of the issue impacting the sex life of your own. This causes it to be simpler to look for a means to fix whatever sexual issue you're experiencing.

## Medication

Various medicines because of the expansion of women's sex drive exist. Just before you think of taking some libido enhancer for women, forever guarantee you consult the doctor of your own. She or he is able to say if the body of your own is able to deal with these enhancers and what type to choose. Several herbs that contain certain ingredients or alkaloids that enhance your libido exist and may be utilized as an all-natural Viagra but before going herbal or maybe orthodox, involve the doctor of your own.

Hormone remedy Hormonal imbalance could be the root cause of reduced libido of women therefore to be able to fix this, physicians put these women on a hormone treatment therapy to increase the various human hormones active in the inciting pleasure for enjoyable and healthy sex. It's essential to allow your physician to suggest what kind of hormone treatment therapy you need to be put on.

## Methods To Help Yourself To Have Much Better Sex Life

The physical transformations the body of your own undergoes as you grow older also have a significant impact on the sexuality of your own. Declining hormone levels as well as changes in circulatory and neurological functioning may result in sexual problems such as for instance vaginal pain or erectile dysfunction.

Such physical changes frequently mean the intensity of youthful sex could give way to far more subdued responses during later life and middle. Though the psychological byproducts of maturity - increased confidence, much better communication skills, and also reduced inhibitions - will help develop a richer, more nuanced, and ultimately fulfilling sexual knowledge. Nevertheless, lots of people fail to understand the complete potential of later life sex. By knowing the essential physical as well as mental elements which underlie satisfying sex, you are able to better navigate problems in case they arise.

Treating sexual issues is easier right now than ever. Groundbreaking medications and expert sex therapists are there in case you need them. But you may be ready to resolve small sexual issues by making a handful of adjustments in the lovemaking style of your own. Allow me to share a few things you are able to try at home.

Prepare yourself. Plenty of great self-help materials are out there for every kind of sexual issue. Browse the web or maybe the local bookstore of your own, choose a couple of energy which pertains to you, and also make use of them to support you and the partner of your own become better educated about the issue. If talking directly is simply too hard, you and the partner of your own is able to underline passages that you especially love and show them to one another.

Try giving yourself time. While you grow older, the sexual responses of your own slow down. You and the partner of your own can improve the chances of your own success by finding a peaceful, comfortable, interruption-free setting for sex. Additionally, realize that the actual physical changes within your body imply that you will require more hours being aroused and reach orgasm. If you consider it, spending more hours having sex is not a bad thing; operating these bodily necessities to the lovemaking routine of your own is able to open up doors to an innovative type of sexual knowledge.

Utilize lubrication. Frequently, the vaginal dryness which starts in perimenopause can be corrected with lubricating gels and liquids. Pick these easily to stay away from very painful sex - an issue which may snowball into flagging libido and growing connection tensions. When lubricants no longer perform, discuss other choices with the doctor of your own.

Maintain actual physical affection. Even in case you are tired, tense, or maybe upset about the issue, engaging in kissing as well as cuddling is crucial for maintaining a physical and emotional bond.

Training touching. The sensate focus methods that sex therapists use will help you re-establish physical intimacy with no feeling pressured. Numerous self-help books as well as informative movies provide variations on these exercises. You might also need to ask the partner of your own to touch you in a fashion that he or maybe she'd love to be touched. This can provide you a much better sense of just how much pressure, from mild to firm, you need to use.

Try out various positions. Establishing a repertoire of various sexual positions not just adds interest to lovemaking, but could additionally help conquer issues. For instance, the improved stimulation to the G-spot which occurs when a man enters the partner of his from behind will help the women reach orgasm.

Jot down the fantasies of your own. This exercise can enable you to explore likely activities you believe may be a turn on for you or the partner of your own. Try thinking of a movie or an experience that aroused you then share the memory of your own with the partner of your own. This is particularly of great help for people with very low desire.

Do Kegel exercises. Both women and men are able to improve the sexual fitness theirs by exercising the pelvic floor muscles of theirs. In order to do these exercises, firm up the muscle you will make use of when you are attempting to quit urine in midstream. Hold the contraction for 2 or perhaps 3 seconds, then release. Do this ten times. Try to do 5 sets one day. These exercises can be accomplished wherever - while driving, sitting at the desk of your own, and standing in a checkout line. At home, women might work with vaginal weights to add muscle mass opposition.

Talk to the doctor of your own or maybe a sex therapist about where you can get these and the way to use them.

Try to relax. Do something relaxing together prior to having sex, like playing a game or even going out for a pleasant dinner. Or perhaps try relaxation strategies such as for instance deep breathing exercises or even yoga.

Make use of a vibrator. This device is able to assist women to learn about their own sexual response and permit her to show the partner of her what she likes.

Do not give up. In case none of your efforts appear to do the job, do not give up hope. The doctor of your own could determine the root cause of the sexual problem of your own and might be equipped to identify treatments that are effective. She or he is able to likewise place you in contact and have a sex therapist who could enable you to explore concerns that could be standing in the form of satisfying sex life.

# FOOD AND HERBS WHICH MAY BOOST WOMEN SEX DRIVE

Sex drives are a finicky idea. Everything out of your menstrual cycle to just how much stress you are under at the office is able to trigger a slight change. But an unexpected change in the libido of your own may also be an indication of an underlying medical problem in several instances (we'll touch on this later).

Here is a roundup of the main foods connected with improving the women libido, together with some backed by hefty investigation and some which might become more folklore than science.

Particular foods, including herbs, are proven to raise sex drive in no less than a couple of studies. Just remember that many of these studies have not been rigorous or big very, and so do not put all your dreams and hopes on them.

Another tidbit to keep in mind with regards to organic supplements: Doses differ from item to item, that make sure you stay within the manufacturer's guidelines.

On that note, it is likewise a good option to check out in with the healthcare provider of your own or maybe a pharmacist about how all of these supplements may interact with:

prescribed medications
over-the-counter medications
vitamins
various other organic supplements

## Ginkgo

Ginkgo biloba is a favorite herbal supplement that may be eaten in numerous forms. Preliminary research indicates that ginkgo may be helpful as an all-natural aphrodisiac.

Nevertheless, the results of research on the usage of ginkgo are inconclusive on if it improves the sexual function of women.

Where you can find it

You are able to purchase ginkgo Biloba in many health food stores or maybe on the internet in the form of:

tablets
capsules
fluid extracts
dried tea or leaves
Ginseng
Searching for another easy-to-find health supplement? Ginseng is one that has numerous possible health advantages.

A little, recently available analysis concluded that ginseng outperformed the placebo to help you fight the sexual dysfunction of individuals using methadone. How will this affect individuals that are not using methadone? More research is required, though it might be well worth a go.

Where you can find it
You are able to purchase ginseng at almost all health food stores and also on the internet in the form of:

raw or fresh ginseng
tablets
capsules
fluid extracts
powder

## Maca

Maca might have some possibility of treating antidepressant-induced sexual dysfunction in postmenopausal women. Additionally, maca has historically been utilized to increase sexual desire and fertility.

While research is promising, a recently available review notes that several of the promises that involve maca can be somewhat overblown.

Where you can find it
You are able to purchase maca at almost all health food stores and also on the internet in the form of:

capsules
fluid extracts

powder
Tribulus Terrestris Another organic dietary supplement that could be helpful for boosting libido is Tribulus Terrestris.

Tribulus Terrestris might be a little tougher to find than several of the other herbs mentioned in this post, so the best bet of your own is purchasing online. It is available in the form of:

capsules
fluid extracts
powder

## Saffron

An expensive and popular spice, saffron is usually advised as an aphrodisiac - and earlier analysis backs it up.
Nevertheless, while this particular study discovered an enhancement in sexual arousal, it didn't notice an enhancement in sexual desire.

Where you can think it is You are able to discover saffron threads in specialty supermarkets or maybe spice stores. You can additionally think it is online, where it is also often obtainable in capsule or powder form.

Red-colored wine Red wine is a commonly recommended aphrodisiac. Along with the other potential benefits of its, a wine that is red might also improve sexual function, based on a 2009 study.

Nevertheless, it is essential to be aware that these findings were self-reported by a tiny sample size. Additionally, various other scientific studies suggest that consuming a lot of alcohol might have a reverse impact on libido, therefore moderation is essential.

## Apples

Truth be told, apples might have an optimistic impact on women's sex drive. One study found that women who consumed an apple one day reported a much better quality of sex life.

While this seems promising, this analysis only indicates a correlation between sexual health and apple consumption. It is not entirely clear if eating apples specifically affects sexual function. Plus, there aren't any other major studies on if apples may boost libido.

## Fenugreek

Fenugreek is an herb used both on food preparation and also as a health supplement. Some research suggests it might help increase libido.

A report concluded that fenugreek might be a highly effective therapy to rise women's sex drive. Nevertheless, the majority of the present exploration of fenugreek covers men's sexual health.

Where you can find it You are able to find fenugreek in supermarkets, online, and spice shops. It is readily available in the form of:

seeds
capsules
fluid extracts

powder

Food with anecdotal evidence While not backed by any proof, these herbs and foods have historically been utilized to increase libido. Many people recommend them. Plus, you probably already have a lot of them in the kitchen of your own, which makes them very easy to try.

## Chocolate

Chocolate is a generally advised aphrodisiac. Nevertheless, in spite of the popularity of its, a 2006 study concluded that chocolate consumption did not have a major distinction on the women's sex drive.

## Coffee

Some people suggest coffee as an aphrodisiac, but - while coffee is able to help boost the mood of yours - there is absolutely no research to allow for the claim.

## Honey

While honey is a great supply of antioxidants, there is no scientific proof that suggests it improves libido.

## Strawberries

Strawberries are another very popular choice which some people swear by, despite a shortage of evidence.

Raw oysters The initial Casanova is believed to have started every day by eating fifty raw oysters. Women and men alike have reported improved sex drive after consuming them. However, there is no proof to allow for these claims.

## Capsaicin

Capsaicin, the active element of chili peppers, offers a number of health advantages, such as improved sex drive.

One particular study did conclude which capsaicin enhanced sexual conduct in men rats, but there is no research that indicates the exact same may be accurate for people.

Saw palmetto While saw palmetto is usually suggested boosting libido in both women and men, there is little evidence to allow for the.

In reality, an organized review concluded the alternative. After taking a look at the information from numerous scientific studies, researchers listed reduced libido as a possible complication of saw palmetto used. Nevertheless, little is thought about saw palmetto use by women.

**Chasteberry**

Chasteberry, likewise referred to as Vitex agnus castus or maybe monk's pepper, is a favorite plant-based product used for a lot of women's reproductive health issues.

While the study indicates that chaste berry might help the signs of premenstrual syndrome, there is simply no scientific proof supporting the potential benefits of it's for women sex drive.

## Figs

Yet another generally suggest aphrodisiac, figs are a rich supply of minerals and vitamins. Though the jury is away on the effect of theirs on libido.

## Bananas

A number of people think bananas are able to increase libido, but once again, there is little scientific evidence to allow for this.

Nevertheless, bananas are a terrific supply of potassium, which helps with testosterone synthesis. While testosterone is normally viewed as a men hormone, women have testosterone, along with decreased testosterone could adversely impact sex drive.

## Potatoes

Potatoes are another very popular aphrodisiac, in spite of the absence of scientific evidence.

Nevertheless, sweet potatoes and both potatoes are filled with potassium, which means they provide exactly the same health advantages as bananas.

Issues to stay away from While it is usually safe to experiment with healthy, food-based aphrodisiacs, there are some dietary supplements you will want to keep away from.

**Yohimbine**

Even with the popularity of theirs, yohimbine (or maybe Yohimbe) supplements are potentially harmful. Not merely can they be blacklisted in a few places, though one study learned that the majority of makes did not tag the quantity of yohimbine properly or maybe list the recognized negative side effects on the label.

Spanish fly is yet another aphrodisiac that should be stayed away from because of its potentially risky side effects. Common unwanted side effects of Spanish fly include problems swallowing, painful urination, vomiting blood, nausea, and blood of the urine.

Remember that the majority of what you are able to find today is not really Spanish fly. In most cases, it is a combination of various other herbs that do not have proven benefits.

Mad honey Different than standard honey, mad honey is contaminated with grayanotoxins. While mad honey has historically been utilized as an aphrodisiac, unwanted side effects are able to consist of dizziness, palpitations, headache, convulsions, vomiting, nausea, and much more.

Bufo toad An element in the potentially dangerous love stone aphrodisiac, in addition to the Chinese medicine chan trusted Source, Bufo toad is yet another aphrodisiac which must be stayed away from. It has been documented to possibly cause hallucinations as well as death.

Some other things to try Searching for other methods to boost the libido of your own? You will find many options for increasing the sex drive of your own beyond the use of medical intervention or aphrodisiacs.

Get enough sleep Sleep is extremely essential for the health of your own - such as the sex drive of your own. One particular study suggested that long sleep length was correlated with stronger sexual desire the following day amongst women.
An additional analysis emphasized the relationship between sexual function and sleep quality, concluding that shorter sleep length as well as insomnia were each related to reduced sexual function.

With regards to boosting the libido of your own, getting plenty of sleep is a terrific first step.

Reduce the stress levels Stress of your own is able to have a damaging effect on a lot of aspects of the health of your own, including the sex drive of your own. A recently available analysis discovered a correlation between job stress and women's sexual dissatisfaction, which means any additional stress might be decreasing the libido of your own.

Taking active steps to lower the stress levels of your own might help boost the sex drive of your own.

Check the medications of your own Certain medications might have an impact on your sex drive too. StudiesTrusted Source claims that antidepressants might be connected to reduced sexual desire.

When you are taking antidepressants and also have poor libido, talk to the doctor of your own about just how you are able to deal with any possible side effects. You might even be equipped to adjust the dosage of your own. Simply make certain you do not quit taking them while not speaking with your healthcare provider initially.

## Exercise

Exercise is an excellent way to boost the libido of your own. One study concluded that strength training could improve the excitement and desire sexual of women with polycystic ovary syndrome (PCOS).

Plus, exercise is a good way to minimize stress, which we know can help boost the sex drive of your own.

## Acupuncture

While extra analysis is required, a 2008 review concluded that acupuncture might be a possible way of improving the sex drive of women.

Additionally, acupuncture might help reduce insomnia, stress, and anxiety, all of that may be underlying causes of a drop in the libido of your own.

In case you are more or less not prepared to try out acupuncture, massage is a good alternative. A 2008 study demonstrated that merely touching the partner of your own is able to help reduce stress, signifying a fast massage might help boost the libido of your own.

Practice mindfulness Believe it or perhaps not, learning how to be careful and present might have a significant impact on the sex drive of your own.

Mindfulness is a fantastic tool for reducing anxiety, and investigation indicates that mindfulness therapy greatly improves the sexual desire of women.

Try out yoga Yoga provides countless advantages, and improving the sex life of your own might be one of them.

A 2010 study concluded that twelve days of yoga practice lead to substantial improvement in all of the aspects of the Women Sexual Function Index. Areas measured provided desire, satisfaction, orgasm, lubrication, arousal, and pain during sexual activity.

Try including these yoga moves to your typical yoga practice to enable you to reduce emotional stress and also increase the libido of your own. You are able to also have your partner involved, as well.

When you should visit a physician While fluctuations in the libido of your own are completely normal, think about talking to the healthcare provider of your own or maybe a sex therapist if it gets a continuing issue.

The American Association of Sexuality Educators, Counselors, and Therapists (AASECT) offers a national directory of suppliers.

You will be working with a hypoactive sexual desire disorder (HSDD), now recognized as a woman sexual interest/arousal disorder. It is able to impact anyone, and it might be an indication of an underlying medical problem.

Typical symptoms and signs of HSDD include:

little to no interest in activity that is sexual
seldom having sexual fantasies or thoughts
disinterest in activity that is sexual
lack of pleasure out of sexual activity

## IDEAS TO BOOST YOUR SEX LIFE

Whether or not the issue is small or big, you will find lots of things you are able to do for getting your sex life back on course. The sexual well-being of your own goes hand in hand with your general psychological, physical, and mental health. Talking with the partner of your own, keeping a proper lifestyle, availing yourself of several of the countless fantastic self-help substances in the marketplace, and simply enjoying themselves is able to enable you to weather times that are tough.

Sex. The term is able to evoke a kaleidoscope of feelings. From tenderness, excitement, and love to longing, anxiety, and frustration - the reactions are as diverse as sexual encounters themselves. What is more often, lots of individuals are going to encounter all many others and these emotions in the course of a sex life spanning many years.

**But what's sex, truly?**

On a single level, sex is merely an additional hormone-driven physical feature designed to perpetuate the species. Obviously, that narrow perspective underestimates the intricacy of the human sexual effect. Along with the biochemical forces at your workplace, the experiences of your own as well as expectations help shape the sexuality of your own. The understanding of your own of your own self to be a sexual being, the thoughts of your own about what constitutes a gratifying sexual connection, and the relationship of your own with the partner of your own are factors that are key in the ability of your own to create as well as keep a satisfying sex life.

Speaking with the partner of your own Many couples think it is hard to chat about sex even under the very best of situations. When sexual issues occur, thoughts of hurt, guilt, shame, and even resentment is able to halt chat entirely. As communication that is good is a cornerstone of a great relationship, starting a dialogue is the initial step not only too much better sex life, but additionally to a closer psychological bond. Allow me to share some suggestions for tackling this very sensitive subject.

Get the perfect time to talk. You will find 2 kinds of sexual conversations: the people you're in the bedroom and also the ones you've everywhere else. it is absolutely acceptable to tell the partner of your own what feels great during lovemaking, though It is better to hold back until you are in a basic setting to talk about bigger problems, like mismatched sexual desire or maybe orgasm problems.

Stay away from criticizing. Couch ideas in positive terms, like, I simply like it if you touch the hair of mine lightly that way, instead of concentrating on the negatives. Approach a sexual problem as an issue to be solved collectively instead of a workout in assigning blame.

Confide in the partner of your own about changes in the body of your own. When hot flashes are keeping you up during the night or maybe menopause makes the vagina of your own dry looking, speak with the partner of your own about these issues. It is better he knows what is truly happening instead of interpreting these bodily changes as not enough interest. Similarly, in case you are men and also you don't purchase an erection only coming from the notion of sex, show the partner of your own how to promote you rather than make her feel she is not attractive adequate to arouse you any longer.

Be truthful. You might feel you are protecting your partner's feelings by faking an orgasm, but actually you are beginning down a slippery slope. As difficult as it's talking about any sexual issue, the difficulty level skyrockets after the matter is placed under many years of lies, injured, and resentment.

Do not equate like with sexual performance Create an ambiance of caring and also tenderness; kiss and touch frequently. Do not blame yourself or the partner of your own for the sexual difficulties of your own. Concentrate instead on maintaining physical and emotional intimacy in the relationship of your own. For more mature couples, another likely sensitive topic that is really worth discussing is what'll happen after one partner gives out. In couples that like a proper sex life, the surviving partner will probably prefer to look for a brand new partner. Revealing the openness of your own to that chance while you're both still alive may relieve guilt and think of the procedure easier for the surviving partner later on.

Utilizing self-help strategies Treating sexual issues is easier right now than ever. Groundbreaking medications and expert sex therapists are there in case you need them. But you may be ready to resolve small sexual issues by making a handful of adjustments in the lovemaking style of your own. Allow me to share a few things you are able to try at home.

Prepare yourself. Plenty of great self-help materials are out there for every kind of sexual issue. Browse the web or maybe the local bookstore of your own, choose a couple of energy which pertains to you, and also make use of them to support you and the partner of your own become better educated about the issue. If talking directly is simply too hard, you and the partner of your own is able to underline passages that you especially love and show them to one another.

Security issues as well as the Internet make use of the Internet is an invaluable cause of all information types, like other products and books (such as sex toys) which can improve the sex life of your own. Even though it might be apparent, do not make use of your workplace pc to do such queries, to stay away from possible embarrassment with the employer of your own, who's likely in a position to observe the search history of your own. Individuals that feel uneasy also about making use of the home computers of theirs as well as credit cards to get sex-related info or maybe products on the internet may have the ability to locate a close-by shop (especially in major cities) and also spend with money.

Try giving yourself time. While you grow older, the sexual responses of your own slow down. You and the partner of your own can improve the chances of your own success by finding a peaceful, comfortable, interruption-free setting for sex. Additionally, realize that the actual physical changes within your body imply that you will require more hours being aroused and reach orgasm. If you consider it, spending more hours having sex is not a bad thing; operating these bodily necessities to the lovemaking routine of your own is able to open up doors to an innovative type of sexual knowledge.

Utilize lubrication. Frequently, the vaginal dryness which starts in perimenopause can be corrected with lubricating gels and liquids. Pick these easily to stay away from very painful sex - an issue which may snowball into flagging libido and growing connection tensions. When lubricants no longer perform, discuss other choices with the doctor of your own.

Maintain actual physical affection. Even in case you are tired, tense, or maybe upset about the issue, engaging in kissing as well as cuddling is crucial for maintaining a physical and emotional bond.

Training touching. The sensate focus methods that sex therapists use will help you re-establish physical intimacy with no feeling pressured. Numerous self-help books as well as informative movies provide variations on these exercises. You might also need to ask the partner of your own to touch you in a fashion that he or maybe she'd love to be touched. This can provide you a much better sense of just how much pressure, from mild to firm, you need to use.

Try out various positions. Establishing a repertoire of various sexual positions not just adds interest to lovemaking, but could additionally help conquer issues. For instance, the improved stimulation to the G-spot which occurs when a man enters the partner of his from behind will help the women reach orgasm.

## The G-spot
Grafenberg spot, or the G-spot, named after the gynecologist that initially identified it, is a mound of super-sensitive spongelike tissue situated inside the top of the vagina, just within the entry. Appropriate stimulation of the G-spot is able to produce extreme orgasms. Due to the difficult-to-reach location of its and also the reality that it's most effectively stimulated physically, the G-spot isn't routinely activated for many women during vaginal intercourse. While this has led some skeptics to

question the existence of its, studies have shown that an alternative tissue type does are present in this specific place.

You should be sexually aroused to have the ability to locate the G-spot of your own. In order to think it is, test massaging the finger of your own in a beckoning movement around the top of the vagina of your own while you are in a sitting or squatting position, and have your partner massage the top surface area of your respective vagina until you see an especially vulnerable region. Some women tend to be sensitive and will discover the spot easily, but for other people it is hard.

In case you cannot easily find it, you should not care. During intercourse, most women believe that the G spot can be most quickly stimulated once the men enter from behind. For couples dealing with erection troubles, play regarding the G spot is usually an optimistic addition to lovemaking.

Oral stimulation of the clitoris mixed with hand-operated stimulation of the G spot is able to provide women a very intense orgasm.

Jot down the fantasies of your own. This exercise can enable you to explore likely activities you believe may be a turn on for you or the partner of your own. Try thinking of a movie or an experience that aroused you then share the memory of your own with the partner of your own. This is particularly of great help for people with very low desire.

Do Kegel exercises. Both women and men are able to improve the sexual fitness theirs by exercising the pelvic floor muscles of theirs. In order to do these exercises, firm up the muscle you will make use of when you are attempting to quit urine in midstream. Hold the contraction for 2 or perhaps 3 seconds, then release. Do this ten times. Try to do 5 sets one day. These exercises can be accomplished wherever - while driving, sitting at the desk of your own, and standing in a checkout line. At home, women might work with vaginal weights to add muscle mass opposition. Talk to the doctor of your own or maybe a sex therapist about where you can get these and the way to use them.

Try to relax. Do something relaxing together prior to having sex, like playing a game or even going out for a pleasant dinner. Or perhaps try relaxation strategies such as for instance deep breathing exercises or even yoga.

Make use of a vibrator. This device is able to assist women to learn about their own sexual response and permit her to show the partner of her what she likes.

Do not give up. In case none of your efforts appear to do the job, do not give up hope. The doctor of your own could determine the root cause of the sexual problem of your own and might be equipped to identify treatments that are effective. She or he is able to likewise place you in contact and have a sex therapist who could enable you to explore concerns that could be standing in the form of a satisfying sex life.

To maintain health which is good that The sexual well-being of your own goes hand in hand with your general psychological, physical, and mental health. Thus, exactly the same healthy habits you depend on to keep the body of your own fit may also shape up the sex life of your own.

Physical exercise, exercise, exercise Physical exercise is first and foremost of all the healthy behaviors that could enhance the sexual functioning of your own. As bodily arousal depends greatly on effective blood circulation, cardiovascular exercise (which strengthens the heart of your own as well as blood vessels) is essential. And exercise has a wealth of some other health advantages, from staving off some forms, osteoporosis, and heart disease of cancer to improving the mood of your own and assisting you to get a much better night 's sleep. Additionally, do not forget to add in strength training.

Do not smoke. Smoking plays a role in peripheral vascular disease, that impacts blood circulation to vaginal tissues, clitoris, and the penis. Additionally, women who smoke have a tendency to go through menopause 2 years earlier compared to the nonsmoking counterparts of theirs. In case you are needing assistance quitting, try nicotine gum or maybe patches or maybe question the doctor of your own about the medications bupropion (Zyban) or perhaps varenicline (Chantix).

Make use of alcohol in moderation. Several men with erectile dysfunction discover that having a single drink is able to assist them to unwind, but heavy use of alcoholic beverages is able to make things even worse. Alcohol is able to inhibit sexual reflexes by dulling the main nervous system. Drinking considerable amounts with a long period is able to harm the liver, resulting in an increase in the estrogen generation of men. In women, alcohol is able to cause hot flashes and interrupt sleep, compounding issues currently contained in menopause.

Eat well. Overindulgence in oily foods causes higher blood cholesterol as well as obesity - both the main risk factors for cardiovascular disease. Additionally, being obese can market lethargy along with a bad body image. Increased libido is normally an additional advantage of losing those additional pounds.

Use it and lose it. When estrogen drops for menopause, the vaginal walls shed several of the elasticity of theirs. You are able to slow this process or perhaps reverse it by sexual activity. in case of intercourse is not an alternative, masturbation is as highly effective, though for women, This is best when you utilize a vibrator or maybe dildo (an object resembling a penis) to help you stretch the vagina. For men, long stretches without an erection is able to deprive the penis of a percentage of the oxygen-rich blood it needs to keep good sexual functioning. As an outcome, something comparable to scar tissue develops in muscle cells, which disrupts the capability of the penis to grow when blood circulation is increased.

Putting the fun back to sex Even in the very best relationship, sex could become ho-hum after a selection of years. With a small amount of imagination, you are able to rekindle the spark.

Be daring. Perhaps you have never ever had sex on the family room floor or even in a secluded area in the woods; right now could be the time period to check it out. Or try exploring erotic films and books. Simply the sensation of naughtiness you receive from renting an X rated video could make you feel frisky.

Be sensual. Create a world for lovemaking that is attractive to all 5 of the senses of your own. Focus on the sense of silk against the skin of your own, the beat of a jazz tune, the perfumed fragrance of plants across the area, the gentle focus of candlelight, and also the flavor of ripe, juicy fruit. Pick this heightened sensual attention when making love to the partner of your own.

Be playful. Try leaving like notes into your partner's pocket for her or him to look for later on. Have a bubble bath together - the warm comfortable feeling you've if you leave the tub is usually an excellent lead into sex. Tickle. Laugh.

Be creative. Grow the sexual repertoire of your own and vary the scripts of your own. For instance, in case you are accustomed to making love on Saturday evening, pick Sunday morning instead. Test out new activities and positions. Try sexy lingerie and sex toys in case you won't ever have before.

Be romantic Read poetry to one another under a tree on a hillside. Surprise one another with flowers when it is not a unique event. Plan one day when all you are doing is lie in bed, conversation, and be personal. The most significant tool you've at the disposal of your own is the attitude of your own about sexuality. Armed with information that is good and a good outlook, you will be ready to maintain a proper sex life for numerous years to come.

# Blank Page

# The Definitive Sex Guide for Men

## How to Improve Your Sexual Techniques, Attract Women and Be the Best Lover

Copyright © 2019 by Samantha May

terms of inattention or otherwise, by any usage or abuse of any policies, processes, or directions contained within is the solitary and utter responsibility of the recipient reader.
Under no circumstances will any legal responsibility or blame be held against the publisher for any reparation, damages, or monetary loss due to the information herein, either directly or indirectly.

Respective authors own all copyrights not held by the publisher.

The information herein is offered for informational purposes solely, and is universal as so. The presentation of the information is without contract or any type of guarantee assurance.

The trademarks that are used are without any consent, and the publication of the trademark is without permission or backing by the trademark owner. All trademarks and brands within this book are for clarifying purposes only and are the owned by the owners themselves, not affiliated with this document.

## WHAT YOU NEED TO KNOW ABOUT SEXUAL TECHNIQUES

Sexual techniques don't always mean to do supertrics in bed. Much love happens before sexual intercourse begins.Some people have a very rare and unusual skill level. It reflects an individual's talent to provide a pleasurable experience through sexual intercourse with others, regardless of gender or even race.

For a man, the effectiveness of his sexual performance can be measured as his sexual partner satisfies his sex. Sexual performance is important for both men and women. Men, however, feel deeper of pride when they think or know that their sexual partner is satisfied with their sexual performance.

**Wellness and healthy sex life**

If you think that health is not just health, then you are wrong. Everything is connected. The importance of pen health cannot be denied, but this health is the result of the overall mobility of the body. Satisfactory sexual performance also requires a great deal of endurance. The result of this stability is to keep the body fit and healthy. Wellness indicates a body that works optimally. It also has a psychological dimension. It also applies to the body, which is emotionally healthy.

Staying in shape will also help you be more comfortable with your body and its sexuality. The level of fitness varies from person to person and there is no common standard that everyone should maintain. Maintaining high quality fitness will help you enjoy better sex. It will help protect you from conditions such as obesity that cause other sexual dysfunction.

## Improve sexual performance and confidence with different techniques

Some techniques can be used to increase sexual performance and confidence. Some of these techniques have been used to improve sexual performance. These techniques are aimed at releasing the mind from negative thoughts and eliminating stress from the body.

### Meditation

Reflection helps to increase confidence, concentration and sexual performance. It purifies the mind and tries to get rid of rejection in the body. It is important that efficiency is regularly taken into account.

## Vizualizace

This technique involves presenting a particular case and step-by-step progress. You can imagine a stressful story that is expected of you to the smallest detail. What it does is that the stress, anxiety and anxiety that come with it gradually and gradually decrease. If actions repeat and repeat in your head, you know exactly what you should do when the time comes.

## Tantra

This is an old age practice that helps to formulate spiritual and physical factors in sexual activity. You can do it yourself or with a partner. Tantra practice is a combination of memory and visualization with a new dimension added to each element. Tantra builds on sexual tension and tension, but attracts a person's attention from her genital organs. This helps train the mind and body to improve sexual performance and detect orgasm.

## SEX TECHNIQUES AND SEX EXPLORATION PLAY WITH YOUR LOVER

Men are not ideal female lovers. Not only do they orgasm too easily, but men rarely appreciate what drives women emotionally or how women stimulate themselves to orgasm. Yet few couples are discussing ways to improve their love. We assume that only older generations had an 'under the front' approach to sex. But where are all the liberated couples today willing to discuss the sexual activities that help them bring variety into their sex lives? Most people see sex as a personal and emotional experience rather than a variety of sexual techniques.

The small minority who have an active interest in sex often assume that everyone is sexually insatiable. As if we all think of sex the same way. But we don't. Nor should we do so in a healthy and balanced society. Some people are much more sexually active and respond faster than others. In a competitive world, 'more' is always equated with 'better'. Still, there is no evidence that the high sexes are happier than people with little sexual drive.

There is no such thing as 'normal'. Nor is it 'ideal' for us to have an 'average' libido, like the disadvantage of a low or high urge. We are naturally satisfied according to our sexual appetite.

In the first years of engagement, it is hoped that the little passion will leave a room for discussion! And for many couples, sex is still an understandable part of their relationship that they never discussed. It is useful for other couples to adopt a clearer approach over time in relation to sexual pleasure. Heterosexual people usually engage with sexual orchids between men and people;

Every orgasm I ever had, whether alone or with a loving person, I mean that I'm lying on my stomach with my eyes closed. As I masturbating, my intense focus on the fantasy that releases sexual release is very different from the top of the lover that lasts longer. With a boy, I must focus on the feeling of penetration (the sexual intercourse with clitoral stimulation). Fisting encourages the vagina in the vagina and she can highlight a particular woman. I masturbate through my hips to move rhythmically, but with a girl I'm quite calm.

Of course, the excuse of recommending sexual techniques to whole strangers. If a woman hopes to take advantage of my conclusions, she must recognize with my experiences, including her own enthusiasm to discover three fame and his orgasm through masturbation. Couples need a strong relationship to talk openly about sexual choices.

If you read this sex beginner for men, it may be fair to say that you intend to be a good lover. It is a good start. A man with open access to learning about sex has a great chance to be a great lover.

Here are some important things that you must understand and apply to your sexual techniques.

There are big differences in access to sex between men and women. If you begin to understand these differences, your sexual intercourse technique will improve significantly.

The big difference between couples is the time it takes to reach orgasm. Men can find an orgasm in minutes. It takes women much longer. The worst mistake that a person can make in sex is to assume that their partner needs the same amount of time to get an orgasm. It pays again. It takes women longer to reach orgasm. Sometimes much longer.

The simple reason for a longer orgasm in women is the difference between anatomy and physiology. Men can not understand. But men who understand this can skilfully use this knowledge to become the friend of the women

So how do you give an orgasm to a woman who wants to remember her?

Understand how you can give a lot of pre-recorded to her. Talk here and ask what she likes. Her erogenous belts include her nipples and her boobs. Ask her if she likes to caress them.

Take your time with your foreplay. And you can pretend the words you use, yourself and your point of view. This is a favorite sex technique. Add to the sexual tension with the preliminary work. Then relax for a moment. Change the sexual tension with more proactive and then relax again. Repeat this. Then you focus on satisfying a clitoris. An orgasm blowing mind leads to the construction of sexual pleasure which is slow but sure.

This beginner sex is an introduction to men being a good lover. And here's another sexual technique that you are not taught at school. Treat her as a sexual goddess that you like and she can be a head.

is the best way to have more sex and your wife to rely entirely on your love than giving her good sex? That's true ... you need to do to keep your wife's sex drive to play and bring peace to ORGASMS every time you bring it to the bedroom it.

Many men, on the other hand, do not give their incredible sex pleasures to their ladies and orgasms are spreading out during sex. Such women are likely to do the following because they are not happy in the bedroom:

- Imagine other men
- Stop trying to have sex with their men because it's so boring
- CHEAT on her husband

With all that, I am willing to give a bet that gives you more sexual pleasure and powerful orgasms for your wife. Am I right? It's good.

## SEXUAL TECHNIQUES THAT EACH HUSBAND SHOULD BRING SEXUAL PLEASURES AND POWERFUL ORGASMS TO HIS WIFE

### 1. Significant oral sex

Many women told me that most men give oral sex. So there are some tips to give to your wife BIG MAX ...

- Be enthusiastic and make a noise (a woman really turns on this)

- Do not just go for clitoris for wives ... start with their outer label to licking, then vagina and her clitoris to licking when she is very wet

- Find out what is the best move for your wife. Try the clitoris to licking back and forth and up and down and see which is the best corresponding. Change speed and pressure for movements too.

## 2. Deep Spot Method

FINGERING powerful technique is Deep Spot method you can give your wife a vaginal orgasm (only a vaginal orgasm at 30% of women).


Here's how:

- Leave your wife on her back with her legs open

- Enter the centerpiece as far as possible in its vagina

- Head wall to the vagina to stimulate movement "come here".

Do this well and shake, scratch and throw her way through the most powerful orgasm of her life. Period.

### 3. The orgasm of the combination

This is extremely exciting for your wife. Simply use the favorite ORAL technique and the Deep Spot method at the same time.

The combination of both techniques at the same time brings incredible bliss to your wife. Guaranteed.

There are a lot of counseling and sexual techniques that men can try or apply to themselves to try to catch. Treatment of PE or premature ejaculation can be an easy adviser explaining why PE occurs. This confirms the couple that this is normal for men. Then the counselor can suggest some techniques that can help postpone ejaculation.

The stop-starter method is one of these techniques or exercises. In short, a man gets sexual stimulation or encourages him to admit he is about to expel him. The next step is to stop the stimulus for 30 seconds. After this short break, she may continue having sex. This process is repeated until one is ready and willing to ejaculate.

Another method of pressing is provided. Men will again have a sexual stimulus until they feel they are about to avoid it. Once the man feels he is about to come, he or her partner gently squeezes his head for a few seconds. Sexual stimulation is repeated for about 30 seconds and then again. This exercise may be repeated several times until the man is ready for ejaculation.

It is great for men to practice these exercises to improve blood circulation and increase blood flow in erectile tissue. If erectile tissue can be encouraged to have a larger volume of blood than it is used for, it should lead to more. Not only can thicker structures do this, but you also have more control over penis muscles and, of course, delayed ejaculation time.

Counseling and psychosexual therapy have very good results and allow individuals to open up and understand them. This type of therapy gives patients a way to help with their disorders. It allows patients to be honest and solve their own uncertainties. Psychosexual therapy seeks to gain a broad perspective by examining the basics of the patient's stress and anxiety that may arise as a result of non-sexual activities.

There are many options for a man who is interested in his sexual experience or lack. Remember, the average man only takes two to three minutes after entering. So if you're a man and you think you're coming too early, pay attention to the facts. You don't have to be like "par par" as you think.

## Dominance

Women wanted to see who the manager was. It's an animal comedy that returns to the cave days. They like to throw and instruct you to do things. If you haven't tried it, I promise you will like it. Start with the simple task of going to your knee. Then do what you want.

## Diversity

In the bedroom you have to mix things together. There are an infinite number of sexual posts. That's the one you couldn't try. Put her in front of you and come here to sit on her arms. It's called the X location. It's a strange angle of penetration and gives an interesting picture.

## Tease

The best way to tighten it is to harass it when you're not even in the bedroom. I recently went home late at night with my boyfriend. I pressed her against the wall and left with her. Then I put my hands in her panties. I have been encouraging her for centuries, but just before she stopped. She was very excited, but very horny. Of course we had a lot of fun at home.

It is a great pleasure to make time and place. Just turn it and then stop it. Then again. It's amazing

## SET YOUR BEDROOM ON FIRE WITH THESE THREE SUPER HOT SEXUAL TECHNIQUES

Is your sex life the same ordinary, last routine?

I understand how you feel and you have to understand that this is a case that affects every couple. We do routine and using elegant nights is difficult. When your relationship is normal, you must be willing to take the next step.

Sadly, how many relationships are breaking up and that are breaking up because of sex. Women, this is a problem that can be easily solved. It is true that you might think that your husband is happy, but he can play moves. In fact, most men are willing to make direct contact with the skin, but it can be boring.

So I'll give you three techniques to swear that your husband will be safer and more than you have long seen. While these people guarantee that your husband will be happy, I also promise a smile from ear to ear.

We all know how fresh the shower is in the morning, revived us and we feel alive. I'm not telling you that you have sex in the shower, which would be normal. I want to bring the shower when it waits, and put it very well and then leave it in the bath.

Now you cross it and rhythmically manage it as fast as you can. Between the scent of soap and hot water that hits your body, it will be an exciting experience. Another advantage is that women lead the story and love men. If you remember an orgasm for a while, you can really masturbate while you shower. This will also have a visual impact that people love.

**Find out the megaphone**

Variable or shout? Whatever you are, I think you're not cut out enough for your husband. Men want to hear how they give you and combine moans and shouts with joy. So even if you are a silent type, notice that you have some noise. Also tell your husband how he feels and tell him when he meets the perfect place. The more aggressive you are, the more sexually aggressive. It can be a key experience, so your ban is released and forget what the neighbors say!

## Think about high school

I think that most of us remember our first sexual experience in the back of the car seat. For me, good memories are always back. Of course, the situation is not always comfortable, but is very close. Turn the radio over and cover the windows. And as long as you do, you don't ask anyone to come to the car. So don't let your husband push you out tonight and make you a back seat outsider.

You will love the way hard space has to move your bodies much closer together. Be sure to choose a slightly distant location!

you don't have to go big to restore passion in your sex life. They are three very simple but very sensual techniques that will ignite the flame you have lost. So try one or try everything and see what happens to your sex life and your love life.

I bet two people will feel trapped for a while.

The most important thing you can do is take control of the story and give your husband what he wants and wants. Stop thinking like a woman and think like your man.

Sometimes it can be difficult to satisfy many women from bed to bed. This did not prevent the boys from trying to be in bed well.

Trying to give love to a woman is a kind of pleasure that makes them completely crazy. Some men try to apply all the leisure techniques they read from a sexual guide to their wives. Many people are surprised when their new skills are over.

These boys do not understand that great sex is always unconscious and is neither logical nor rational. Too hard to focus on technology, such as the exact pressure or angle of your hand, the direction of your rhythm, or the "right" set of actions, can hinder sex satisfaction.

This is because no matter how much training you have received, two women do not respond in the same way in a certain way, and the same woman may have different responses on different occasions. Controlling specific maneuvers is therefore a future exercise if you do not understand this important fact of the sexuality of women.

Any man can learn the technique from a self-help book. However, this does not discriminate in any way. You have to give her what no one else can do. Your attention is the secret component of the best technology that can bring a woman to nature. To master this technique, you must learn the important principle of this: NOTE

I want to pay attention to this. Pay attention to her body. In addition to the bright spots - the clitoris and the G-point - take the time to explore them and contact other potential hot spots, such as ears, neck, lower back, buttocks, knees and legs to see where it has its own hot spots .

You do this by paying attention to what it says, how it cools, how it looks and looks, how it moves, and how its skin structure changes. You must be aware of your feelings and emotions. To see this, use the five senses: sound (ears), sight (eyes), touch (hands), smell (nose), taste (tongue). In fact, this is the best advice about sex that can be applied to any woman.

There are many reasons why this approach is so strong:

**(1) Every woman is different**

One of the reasons for the failure of "technology" is that each woman is different and work does not work with one woman for another. But what works for every woman is cautious. By comparing how she responds to your headphones and sexual contact, you can see exactly where she likes and whether she needs it slowly or fast, hard or smooth. , temporarily or immediately.

## (2) Increase your sexual confidence

There is nothing more than a woman or a man who is sexually confident - a man who knows exactly what he is doing and is not careful, shy, insecure, or cares about his sexuality. Being deeply involved in your body as it travels, succeeds and breathes, you will be too busy thinking about your insomnia, shame, or fear of sex. Then you will find her as a sexually confident man. Another benefit is that you are also excited by sexual reactions.

## (3) It has a close relationship and attachment

The strongest sexual organ in a woman's body is not between her legs. He's in his head. When a woman feels confident and joins her husband, she can surrender completely to you. When this happens, she is able to experience orgasms that are much stronger than anything she ever had. He may not realize that he can attain such a level of joy.

When you master the art of care, it begins to feel that close relationship with your attention. It will focus on you and your body. This coordination acts as a bridge between sex and passionate love. When he enters this emotional state, he gains the strongest sexual experience of his life…

**SUPERMAN ENDURANCE DURING SEX - DESTROY HER FURIOUSLY WITH THESE MURDEROUS SEXUAL TECHNIQUES!**

Anyone who wants in this world (except the Dalai Lama) needs perseverance that will satisfy women in bed. You will see that it is difficult to keep a long-term woman unless you have sexual stamina ... if you stay in the bedroom for only 2 minutes, no woman would want to stay with you. It's sad, I know, but that's true!

But don't worry ... there's a help. You can easily develop long-term endurance by following the techniques I would like to share with you here. Read on to find out the ways of murder that "maintain distance" in terms of satisfying and satisfying a woman during sex ...

Superman's Sexual Durability - With these sexual murder techniques it destroys fun!

"The Art of Interruption". Make a list of all the sexual tasks you know and master - dog style, courageous missions, backstopping, or even Kenny Geylow's famous status. Then find out which pages are usually the first. Then launch the sexual site you are sensitive to, and then change regularly. This gives you some control, so you won't succeed quickly.

"Double condom". Buy two banks in different sizes. Then throw both things! This would disassemble the pipe and would have a better ability to control your ejaculation. If you change quickly and wear double condoms, you must create a female orgasm before doing so.

**Here's how to send her into orgasms - Here's a BIG read book about incredible sexual techniques! Read this**

So you had partners. Or a partner. Do you know how to send her orgasms? Have you ever experienced that great feeling when your partner's face turns red, becomes completely stiff and then relaxes when he has a screaming orgasm, involuntary convulsions and is apparently in a state of maximum ecstasy? No? Then you miss so much. It is the original sense of victory. But don't worry - you send a girl with screaming orgasms.

The trick in managing a partner in orgasm is to know the different dimensions needed for a female orgasm. In men, sex is 80% physical and 20% psychological. In women it is 60% physical and 40% psychological. You thought I'd say "for women it's 20% physical and 80 psychological", right?

This is the nonsense of the "new age" that so many men buy. They believe that telling your partners how much they love them will bring them into smoking orgasms. It can help - but by no means will it cause an orgasm!

**Psychological**

They must be in the right mood. And the "real mood" varies from woman to woman. Some women prefer a good old mood of "weak light - soft music and sensual lovemaking", while a growing number of other women prefer a "rough, quick kitchen in the kitchen" or a variant of spontaneous sex. Whatever it is, learn it. No one in the world can say what your women liked most. You have to find it. Only a query can do a good position!

## Physically - that's how you send her to orgasms

The physical part is more difficult, but you just need to do it. The first thing to keep in mind is not to challenge it until it's finished. This is, like the last GOLD rule of sending women into orgasms that most men do not understand. To make sure your penis fits properly, it must be ready.

In fact, it should be more than ready. Once wet, it may look like it's done, but as I said, go over and over. You should let her beg for it.

That's an incredible way to get her into wild orgasms, believe me. She will beg, the thought that your penis is in her will make her crazy and crazy every minute she asks for it; and when you finally put your penis in it, it will look like it's in heaven!

There are many sexual techniques that we can use to satisfy our women. Think about it, think about it - every week we could read men's magazines and internet books and find countless techniques.

However, many sexual techniques are not very good and do not produce the results we want.

Fortunately for you, I am going to share with you a sex technique that is extremely effective. So if you want a user-friendly technique that works every time ... read it and use this information the next time you want your wife to vote for glowing hot sex.

The sexual technique I want to share with you needs to be used during FOREPLAY.

How to do it ...

When kissing your wife, gently push your hair toward a solid object (the wall is the best choice) and start kissing your hair.

Remember to kiss your wife's body parts that also respond best. Some women like to kiss, fool and lick their ears. Others like it when their husbands bite and gently kiss their necks.

As a husband, your goal should be to find out where and how your wife likes to kiss you.

Have you been with me so far? Great.

Now let's go a little further and talk about the sexual technique you want to use to warm up, moisten and breathe ...

While kissing his wife, gently pull up his shirt, so now there's nothing on her stomach. Do the same with your wife's shirt and press your stomach against her.

Sounds ridiculously simple, doesn't it?

You will notice, however, that as soon as your belly touches, something pretty nice happens - you will find that your wife begins to breathe harder and immediately begins to kiss you passionately.

You will have to agree that this is great because it only takes a few seconds to perform the "T-shirt trick" and yet your wife will now be more sexually aroused, warm, wet and horny than you. usually predicts it in 20 minutes!

I think it is fair to say that the "T-shirt" is the overture of STEROIDS.

And it works every time.Before you try, there are a few things to remember before you use a trick-shirt.

1. Your wife should not know that you wanted to use this technique. Instead, it should be natural.

In other words, do not pay attention to what you are doing - the first thing you need to know is when your stomach handles it.

2. Another thing you should think about, even if it is a great technique in your "bedroom" - it's just a predictive technique.

In other words, it is only a technique to attract your wife and prepare for the "main course". Of course she will be hot, wet and horny and ready to let her come but won't let her resign ... then you have to use another sexual technique to give the woman the ORGASMS she needs.

Many people believe that sex is one of the most important factors in any relationship. When a woman tries to get sex, expect 100% sexual satisfaction. If you're one of those guys who don't have a real sex technique or breathe too fast, you can't offer it. You are considered to be a very poor lover and can endanger relationships.

One of the biggest mistakes boys make is to think that sex is completely physical. That can't be out of the truth anymore! A woman is a very emotional woman, and therefore emotions play a huge role in her sexual satisfaction. Below are some effective ways to crush all women's ears after sex.

# # 1 Don't rush her

Don't forget to take the time. Never squeeze while having sex. Try to keep things natural and gradually rise. If the rhythm is destroyed, it is difficult to have an orgasm or even sex in general. You have to work on it that wants you to make progress. Try to keep it smooth and whispering in your ear about how good it looks and smells. It's also important to remember that women often love more than sex themselves, so don't play it!

## # 2 Caress Her

Before you jump into sex right away, it's important to spend some time staring at it. This is important to encourage and motivate in advance.

I think it's one of the best places to care for a woman in her thighs. You will get a moan before you know it gently and slowly meet there. When you do, try kissing her passionate kissing. Now for bonus tips!

When you read every single word in this book, the best ways to increase her sexuality will come to the fore and you will discover the exact steps to wake up your loved ones well.

1. You may be smart enough to realize the need to start with a prelude, but you may not know all of its erogenic zones that give it an intense passion. Soft cushions in the neck and shoulders

are a great place to start. If you want to go one step further and use the outer chest and easily draw circles around your finger, prepare the stage for an unforgettable evening. And don't forget her inner thighs, use them to stroke your hands and kiss them gently.

2. Now you know something more about her erogenous zones, about her thoughts. Do you think you should get her in the right mind? If you said yes ... most people prefer it. Women must focus on sex, otherwise they will not enjoy the experience. You know, women are usually consumed by the thoughts and stress of everyday life. They hardly close the outside world and focus only on themselves. So, before you think about sex and pleasure, make sure your mind is in the right place.

3. Maybe you think I would explain some of the best techniques and positions for creating a women's orgasm. I think it is important to take care of the preparatory things before delving into the best sex techniques. And to be honest, the best positions are usually the ones she likes. But if you want to help her have an orgasm ... choose

positions that can stimulate both the clitoris and vagina.

Now I want you to use what you just learned. Use this information to learn how to sexually arouse a woman and become a better lover. Any experienced man who has extended his skills in love knows that lack of sex will never be a problem.

Here are some tips from experts:

- Do not worry, because orgasm is not so important;
- Relax a little more and stop focusing on orgasm;
- Try to accept an adequate amount of leg, abdomen and buttock tension;
- Rhythmically pushed into the floor muscles of the pelican;
- Breathe in or take a deep breath to get oxygen into the tense muscles;
- Close your back or try a different position to maximize clitoral pacing;
- Encourage the lubricating clitoris long enough to guarantee orgasm; and

- Escape your favorite phagos to prevent negative thoughts or distractions!

I am not saying that these approaches do not work. They probably work for the people who represent them. I'm just saying they don't work for me. Yet I thought that female orgasm should happen naturally like men?

Men's experience is simpler and therefore more open to each other in the way they enjoy their sexuality. Women are experiencing more because of a lack of understanding. Women rarely compare notes, even when they are bullied, succeed in transmitting ornamental techniques to sex with a partner.

**Facts about female sexuality**

Most women (including many experts) feel uncomfortable with eroticism and explicit sexual behavior. So, while men know that their PSYCHOLOGICAL sexual arousal depends on an appreciation of eroticism (images of the body of a real or imagined sexual partner), women are told that female sexual arousal simply comes from love and romance.

Although men are aware that they need PHYSICAL stimulation of their penis to experience orgasm, women are told that stimulation of the clitoris is not necessary for female orgasm. The fact is that women should be more SEXUAL than men if they were able to achieve orgasm without using (physical and psychological) orgasm techniques that men do ...

I try to analyze the facts by comparing and contrasting the sexual experiences of men and women. My suggestion is that enjoying our sexuality through sexual arousal and orgasm includes:

obtaining PSYCHOLOGICAL sexual arousal through an appreciation of eroticism (images for men; stories for women); and

(only once sexually aroused) achieve orgasm through PHYSICAL stimulation of the sexual organs (penis for men; clitoris for women).

Experts sometimes suggest that women should use their orgasm techniques (obtained from masturbation) during sex with a partner. With all the stress of clitoral stimulation, it is easy to overlook other important aspects of masturbation.

"Fantasy and masturbation go together like bacon and eggs and many people have a favorite that always guarantees an orgasm. Studies show that more than 50 percent of us fantasize every time we make love to our partner.

When I speak to other women, I know that I have studied my sexuality more than most. I have been masturbating since I was seventeen and I have more than twenty years of regular sexual intercourse, including trying different sexual techniques with my partner. I am glad that if there were magical solutions, we would have found them already.

Sex plays an important role in the relationship. However, few claim to be sexually satisfied in the relationship with which they are associated. This can be caused by physical problems such as erectile dysfunction and premature ejaculation, or simply due to emotional problems. There are even people who think they are weak. This is sad and something regarding the application of tantric sexual principles.

The principles that make up the tantric philosophy of sexual performance have been used for thousands of years. Although originally used only to enhance people's ability to experience joy and happiness, the application of these principles has been extended to all parts of human experience, including the bedroom. People who use these principles in sexual intercourse usually have better sense of gratification and emotional satisfaction. The reason is that the basic principles of all tips on tantric sex work.

One of the basic principles of sexuality is sexual freedom. All tantric sex techniques and tips usually try to exploit couples' spiritual sensuality. The various techniques used are usually designed to eliminate any inhibition that society has created over time, allowing couples to explore the full range of sexual pleasure. This is usually useful for couples to enjoy the sexual energy they share, giving them an increased level of intimacy. Without any inhibition of sex, full pleasure in using tantric sex tips is usually guaranteed.

Tantra principles usually contain sex and emphasize the increased sexual consciousness. Therefore, not only can a person with greater sexual awareness enjoy full sexual, but also keep control of the level of tension so that he can stay as long as he wants. These principles usually provide targeted sexual energy and an intense long-term period of sexual pleasure, allowing long orgasms to broaden the mind.

It is known that tantric techniques only help to overcome their sexual and emotional disorders. This is usually achieved by opening the door to a high compassionate platform, understanding and sexual consciousness. By removing barriers to high sexual performance, these principles usually provide a good platform for long-term close relationships and long-term sexual pleasure.

There is also a complete surrender to the great life of gifts for sexuality. This approach to sex usually causes a man to forget all sexual expectations, which helps him not to fear failure. With less anxiety, a person is usually better to control his ejaculation to help prevent premature ejaculation.

## HOW CAN I PREVENT PREMATURE EJACULATION? SIMPLE SEX TECHNIQUES THAT YOU NEED TO KNOW

Not only your question, but many men have the same question. If you are looking for simple techniques to prevent the problem from eliminating your partner's satisfaction, these tips will help you avoid the problem. You may need to use one of these techniques to overcome the problem, or you may need to collect more than one technique to get the result you want.

One of the best ways to prevent premature ejaculation is to take full control of your mental and emotional situation before and during sexual acts. If you can be responsible for your mental processes, you can focus more on what is happening at the moment, such as sexual sex control.

Physical exercises can be great, but the most important idea is to control the PC muscles that control the movement of sperm in your penis. To do this, you must do the first thing. The PC volume controls ejaculation. And if you can control this muscle, you will have full strength in the long run. This exercise is also a solution, especially if you ask, how can I prevent premature ejaculation?

Try to take different sexual positions. Sexual positions as missionaries are the most popular sex techniques, but they are not effective if you want to prevent premature ejaculation. You can read Kamasutra to experiment with trying other sexual positions. One of the useful sexual positions, and the most recommended by the expert, are women in the highest position. This can help you better control your ejaculation. But you can try a number of other sexual positions based on your creativity.

Many boys are wasting their money on ineffective pills and creams, which are basically unnecessary because they only solve the problem but do not cure it. They also usually have many side effects because they have different types of chemicals. How to avoid early ejaculation is easier than you think. Anyone could do it no matter how bad your condition is. The first stage is to start and use the right technology for you.

There are many ways a person can live longer in bed. All you have to do is find out what really works for him and try to use it to improve the performance of his bedroom. Special features, deep breath and tactically changing sex work are sexual factors that have helped many men stay in bed longer. Here's why and why these methods are effective to help a person delay ejaculation.

There is no intention that the frequency of entering a woman will determine her level of voltage. This is because tension intensity usually increases with increasing stroke frequency due to increased friction between the penis and the vagina. So start with slow banks and reduce their penetration and then increase your bank's pace as your partner becomes more and more. This will ensure that there is no direct increase in sexual energy, which can lead to premature ejaculation. If you want to stay longer in bed, always start.

A great way to stay longer in bed and make sure that his chain of tension is not interrupted is by deep pressure into it, and instead of meeting the body that moves into and out of her vagina, wipe the pelvis across her clit. Clitoral stimulation will help keep them aroused and the rest break will help reduce stress levels. This is because there is no friction, the shaft is less friction on your body, which means you are so excited. This should ensure that you stay in bed longer.

Although the start and stop technique is effective in helping men stay in bed for longer, these are usually challenges when it comes to implementing this technique. This is because the stops can be so difficult that they can break your partner's tension chain. To prevent premature ejaculation while avoiding unpleasant moments, simply change your sexual position when you start. It looks like a natural thing and doesn't reduce the excitement of your partner. The period between changing sexual positions should be sufficient to give you time to relax and help you stay in bed longer.

Fear of failure is a major cause of premature ejaculation. This is because nervousness usually causes great tension in the human body and therefore makes it difficult to control the ejaculation process. If you relax your body by deep breathing during and before sex, you will stay in bed longer because it gives you more control over yourself.

However, all of these sexual techniques should not be used alone if you want to stay in bed longer. You should always use different methods to postpone ejaculation at the same time for better sexual performance.

This is particularly the case since most techniques usually complement each other. It is also good to remember that men are involved differently and what can work for one man to prevent premature ejaculation may not work for another. Therefore, it is recommended to use different methods to stay longer in bed and if you find a way to help you endure as long as you want, be with it. You can always last longer and these methods of delaying ejaculation will certainly help you.

We will discuss the brain element of this section about improving sexual techniques such as loving art. We will also explain why improved love love techniques can give a woman a sexual disorder to overcome any disorder.

First of all, you should know that the following tips do not work for all women, but have been tested and approved by ordinary people around the world for some of the best ways to make love techniques. improvement.

Sexual techniques and techniques consist of love rather than art, and you must be an artist who can master them perfectly. There are many different techniques, so you can try them all and see the ones that are most useful to you.

Techniques are also divided into groups for specific people. For example, if your penis is longer, try another place that allows you to use distance and encourage other parts of the woman's body. If you are not in very good physical condition, try other sites, etc. In short, there are several techniques for each pair.

There are also a number of exercises that can improve your sexual performance. They are directly aimed at better construction and help you to control your penis as much as possible. It is important that during sexual intercourse you control your ejaculation while letting it go as your partner. This is often considered the perfect handle, so Kegel exercises would be tested. You can get a lot of information about the Internet.

Perfect loving techniques also require you to be in good physical condition, especially if you want to practice more advanced techniques. Therefore, I recommend going to the gym at least once a week and it should be good. Remember that a nice body also attracts your partner, even if it doesn't. She probably doesn't know, but her brain is made in such a way that looking at the top-level male body causes sexual intercourse. Her other senses resist it, but a beautifully shaped body helps a lot.


Sexual disorder in women is often associated with poor performance under the layers. We are not suggesting that you are not doing as well as you can, but there is a problem and it is prevented by sex. If you can show her the positive side of sex, she can easily overcome her problem and everything will soon return to normal. Concentrate on your love techniques and make sure they approve and enjoy it. This will help you both better understand and have a nice and very meaningful relationship.

Sexual desire and joy are our primary rights. After all, we are created naked and with different genitals. He had to keep in mind the plan. We are sexual beings from the day we are born to the day we die. Sex is vital to our lives and seems to be an area of life that deeply touches our personal problems. Our sexuality is the basic expression of who we are. We can hide from sex, we can hide from sex, but we cannot be completely sexual and hide.

Why have sex? It is known that sex improves our lives in several ways, both psychologically and physically.

Health benefits include lower blood pressure, overall stress reduction, higher antibody levels, so fewer colds and fleas, calorie burning, good exercise, improving cardiovascular health, enhancing self-confidence, releasing endorphins and reducing physical pain and helping with it. relieving depression; reduces the risk of prostate cancer; promotes sleep.

Personally, good sex is perhaps only 20% of a good relationship (80% if bad), but it's crucial 20%. Orgasm increases the levels of oxytocin, a hormone with which we can feed and bind. Sex therefore increases love and connection on a purely biological basis. Sex is an arena that is special for a couple. We let our sexual partner know in a way we don't share with anyone.

A couple with a satisfactory sex life can build and maintain a long-term love relationship. It is known that people are more stable and productive in their work, have better health and live longer.

The most beneficial sexual experiences are much richer, more varied and creative than the get it method. And sexual sensitivity has nothing to do with being able to meet the prototype of sexual attraction in culture. Rather, it grows from the connection between hearts, ghosts and bodies. Very good sex begins with the willingness to be open and vulnerable and voluntarily bringing joy and value. The psychological ability to share a close relationship, both physically and emotionally, is essential for good sex, but it is an art that confuses and even intimidates many people.

Good sex is therefore good because of openness and confidentiality, risk and control, personal satisfaction and mutual compliance. Good sex requires the ability to be immersed at the moment (which is difficult for most people), always present for human identity, our partner and our life.

In order to maintain a healthy and balanced sex life, we need to pay increased attention to our senses, the physical, emotional, intellectual and spiritual aspects of us and our relationships with our partners. We need to consider ("Know yourself") to know what we want and that we need sexually. Then we have the courage and confidence to express these wishes to our partner, even in the light of possible rejection. We must also give up a series of narcissistic self-confidence that, when we were young, could have prevented us from adapting to the reality and needs of someone else.

What I mean is: good sex requires PSYCHOLOGICAL VALUE (which we all have because we have been living for a while now and have learned a few things on our way.)

Older lovers not only experience satisfying sex, but more often have sexual ecstasy. In sex there may be certain conditions that remove the boundaries of self in relation to the "other". This kind of well, self-transcendence, can open channels and experience the feeling of a wider and more universal connection.

Let's see what the dictionary says about "ecstasy": nice pleasure; intense joy; mental transport or incorporation of considerations of divine things; displacement; trance; the shared feeling that someone will take you or move you from you or your normal state and enter into a state of heightened emotions so strong that transference as a dissociation arises from everything that is the only powerful feeling; this trance or record is associated with a mysterious promotion.

Oriental sexual ecstasy associations regularly coincide with spiritual perspectives. In addition to Western civilizations, there is a gap between sex and God.

It is like that, right? Everything from your blood pressure to lowering mystical heights shows that the good thing is sex.

But if it's so good, why don't you have so much sex? or are they exposed to various sexual dysfunction, debt or danger?

It is a fact that many of us will never use this opportunity to explore every sexual opportunity. One author I read referred to those who achieve sexual compliance as a "blessed couple."

What makes a person good in bed? You had to hear a saying no matter what size you were, but how you used it. This is important for women in bed and men must achieve it. Read on to find out how a woman leads a bed using these simple yet effective techniques.

It's more than just physical - women feel that sex is much more than just physical and orgasm. During the activity, you have to make more emotional contact with them than with anything else. If you know what you're really doing, it doesn't matter.

Be sensitive - it is understood that women are sensitive, but when you are as sensitive as you and enjoy the same way your company enjoys, the pleasure is doubled and you see your partner better and more passion. .

Fantasies - Women love fantasies and nothing can drive them more desert than a man who discusses fantasies and who knows what he needs in bed. Before doing this, discuss and describe each step you want to sleep with. Take a sample of the movie it is watching and put it in the mood. Then act slowly and steadily, but try to keep the finest and slowest way to gain as much passion as possible.

It seems that women who are sexually satisfied are absolutely sweet, more caring and less hopeless. Many people can become uncomfortable if men are not sexually satisfied. He can remain in the constant mood of PMS and can cheat you only because he hopes to find a person with better sexual techniques.

Some women do not give men full enthusiasm if they arise regularly during the peak. It is not clear that women have as much accent as women. You need skills to educate women. Now you can learn the best techniques. Read on and give female orgasms they will never forget!

# 3 Sexual techniques guaranteed to give her the best orgasm in her life

Technique 1: Become a sex machine. Women usually have many more aspirations when they are sexually related than men. To be screaming and sweating, you must be an expert and be creative. Begin your passionate kisses, press harder and make sure they don't fall.

Technique 2: Extension after Dirty Talk. Start telling her how sexy she is. Sexual whispering fantasies in your ear and tell her what you want to do.

During the preview, you can be sure it warms up completely. Every woman likes to have sex, so let her know what she wants to do and whenever she wants to follow your requirements.

Technique 3: Switch to your speed. Use fingers and mouth to stimulate. Keep your personal topline under control as well. Always encourage her, even at rest, to prevent you from finding an orgasm faster than your partner.

There is a lot of ignorance among men about male sexuality. The aim of this section is to destroy some of these male sexuality myths and provide information that men can use to achieve greater sexual satisfaction. Read this book to find out how much you know about male sexuality.

## Men care about their size

Studies show that most men are aware of size. While their body size may be on average with health standards, they may underestimate them and have less confidence in their sexuality. In addition, it has been noted that while many men feel that they are gender-aware because they do not feel able to satisfy them due to the lack of harassment, their partner reports satisfaction with their penis size. According to most women and even sex researchers, the amount of penis is not as important as other aspects such as general sexual well-being, sexual technique and sexual compatibility.

## Men don't always want sex

Contrary to deep-seated beliefs, people do not always want sex. There are times when men wouldn't want to get sex and have no problem. For example. These may be times when men feel too busy or too busy. They can rely on energy and therefore do not have to prove that they desire sex despite the progress of their partner.

## Men can experience more dry orgasms

Like women, men can gain a number of orgasms. However, it may take time and practice before men learn that they have more orgasms. By the way, more orgasms mean you have a number of full-length orgasms or "dry orgasms," so they are different from the type of orgasm most people have. Men can learn that they have more orgasms by learning to control ejaculation and gaining more awareness of their own sexual puzzler.

## Men can control ejaculation, usually if they are not always

According to gender experts, men can achieve the highest level of sexual satisfaction for themselves and their partner by learning to control ejaculation. While most men have problems controlling the ejaculation at some point in their lives, and even some have premature ejaculation, most men do not know that they can control their ejaculation. There are simple techniques and exercises that men with little or no practice can learn to ejaculate and enjoy more sexual pleasure.

## Masturbation is normal and healthy for men

While masturbation was perceived as a danger and a sign of a mental problem, it is now considered a healthy sexual practice for both men and women. Recent studies have suggested that men could reduce the risk of prostate cancer by masturbating regularly. This is because carcinogenic chemicals can accumulate in the prostate if men regularly ejaculate. Because there is a risk of sexually transmitted sexually transmitted diseases, masturbation is a much better option. In addition, sexual temperament and regular orgasms, minimum, stimulates the heart and immune system.

Some sex experts say that masturbation can improve sexual health and relationships. By exploring their own bodies, men can find out what they like sexually and teach their partner motivated. Some couples use mutual masturbation to find techniques to get more satisfying sexual relationships.

**SEX TIP: STAY LONGER IN BED USING TANTRIC SEXUAL TECHNIQUES**
Tantra principles have been used for thousands of years to help people live happily and enjoy the

simple things that make the average person in their daily lives. Sex is one of the most effective tools to explore the limitless limits that can open up the application of tensile principles to human life. With powerful tantric sexuality techniques, a man can prevent premature ejaculation and stay in bed longer. That's why it's possible.

Fear of failure is a major cause of premature ejaculation. Studies show that men who engage in sexual intercourse with less confidence usually do not know the level of tension and rarely have control over the ejaculation process. Therefore, they rarely spend a long time in bed, so they usually cannot sexually satisfy their partners. The reflection system developed according to Tantra's philosophy usually focuses on holistic health and peace for man, which increases man's confidence in the bedroom. A highly effective quantitative approach is also effective in addressing a person's fear of physical and emotional fear that allows him to have a relationship when full.

Every sexual therapist tells you that because of extreme sexual performance, it usually requires a lot of patience, because the slow pace of sexual intensity is caused by the greatest orgasms. Tantra sexual tips usually focus on helping couples manage their responses to sexual stimulation and pay attention to the time to love.

The focus is usually on relationships and not on immediate satisfaction with physical sexual desire. This usually protects many anxieties among men and, of course, helps one to increase his sexual awareness. These principles emphasize the connection between heart, mind, body and soul and provide more intense and longer orgasms.

Most of the problems they encounter when having sexual intercourse are usually caused by condition and emotions, provided that men age. It also includes reduced ability to stay on the long bed, as most men show.

Since tantric sex techniques usually focus on encouraging sensual indigenous human spirituality, the use of sex tips will undoubtedly promote human sexual freedom, thus allowing the free movement of sexual energy during sexual intercourse.

This will play an important role, not only to allow confidence in sexual intercourse, but also to have better overall sexual performance, including building a partner long enough for an orgasm.

In Tantra, this involves identifying sensual indigenous spirituality and encouraging people.

Using these principles one can enter a new world of sexual consciousness, allowing him to find previously suppressed parts of himself. This is mainly because Tantra, in contrast to other sexual tips that focus only on physical sexual satisfaction, emphasizes the connection of man with his body and soul.

In this way, a man can improve his bedroom's sexual performance by using tantra sexual satisfaction techniques. This sexual awareness will also be great to help men stay in bed longer, thus creating effective sexual tools to prevent premature ejaculation.

Sexual freedom is now a matter for most men. This is mainly because of the prohibitions that people develop with aging. It is also due to dozens of concerns and unresolved emotional problems that bring men to the bedroom. It is therefore not surprising that many people have problems with their sex life.

It is one of the main shortcomings of sexual satisfaction in the bedroom because people suffer from erectile dysfunction and other abnormalities such as premature ejaculation

Tantra's reflexive approach has long been refined to ensure that people, especially men, can enjoy parts of themselves, especially sexual intercourse. Tantra includes sex as a friend and does not consider it as bad as some people. Sex is considered a gift of nature and is used and explored across borders. People learn that sex is perfect if his mind, soul and body along with his partners. This usually creates a closer relationship between couples and provides the basis for orgasms and sexual satisfaction. Through increased sexual awareness and sexual freedom, the use of tantric sex techniques provides universal and sexual energy flow between couples. This usually provides deeper levels of relationship and thus great sexual performance.

## LOVE MAKING TECHNIQUES - SEXUAL MISTAKES THAT MOST MEN MAKE

The mistakes I want to share with you are so common that every woman I meet complains. If men stop making all these mistakes, how amazing and fun will their sex life be?

Let me share some common sexual mistakes that men make for you to completely eliminate women:

1. Premature ejaculation. This is where you get to the top of the road too fast for your loving person to be happy. This problem can be solved by techniques. Check out my next book on this topic to learn how to fix it.

2. Lack of predecessor. I'm for prelude. Good foreplay can help increase passion for overall sexual contact. Many men make the mistake of getting too fast for sexual intercourse. Through good and long foreplay you can satisfy your loved ones by being very wet and orgasmic. Believe me, they'll come back to you if you're both on your way later.

3. Too boring. They always use the same old positions and techniques, they feel too predictable. It is therefore important that you continue to learn about new sexual techniques and ideas.

4. Don't eat her enough. Women love to kiss and want to get them when they have sex. Learn the right techniques to kiss and ignore their other erogenous zones.

5. Fall asleep right after sex. This is a very big problem because I got most complaints about it. The study shows that a person usually falls asleep within 3 seconds of sleep. Do not try to clamp if it is not possible. Women want to have fear and love for sex. Tell her how much you love to kiss her and kiss her on the roof and cheeks.

I can assure you that you do not want your mistakes from your relationship, but all of them do.

## Popular forecasting tips and techniques to spice up your sex life

One of the most important challenges and predictive techniques for men with great sex is to remember that a woman usually needs. You could say that the sexual energy of women is like a stove on a stove. It takes a moment for the hot water to enter the bubble.

Most men are now very excited. After a few minutes they usually stand up and can then start intercourse. Therefore, the sexual energy of man is like a flame. It starts quickly, lights up and can show up so quickly.


My best tip for forecast

It is therefore crucial to obtain an orgasm from a woman who will be in the foreplay for a long time. Sexual surveys show that men only spend about 10 minutes in their preparatory work. These studies also show that women attend most male sex techniques as poor and consider themselves better mistresses.

## How to start preparatory work

Focus on connecting with all parts of her body, including toes, fingers, hair, face and legs. If you come in contact with someone you love, make eye contact.

Once your loving person begins to respond to loving contact, you begin to focus on the warmer zones of your body. These include breasts, thighs inside, and finally genitals.

## How to increase energy

Generally, I like spending a lot of time touching, kissing, rotting and breastfeeding my breasts and nipples when it's bigger.

Pay attention to how your wife reacts to contact, and the pleasure of contact with her body should be enjoyed. If you focus on your pleasure, you feel your hand much more fun.

Another term is a prediction that is used to indicate how you both got fired because of an incident. It is the art of perfection in time. He has his own habits and practices; your turn is on each other and you taste each other. The torturers move with each other and give each other satisfying magic; no acceleration of the costs of others; the whole game is the flavor of the last game.

Men are faster and rise very fast on the slope; they are relatively simple, genital contact is often the ultimate sight. There would be a number of recommendations for a woman. Attack her for a long time before placing her on the bed. Look at it in your quest, undress it and mind with these movements. Let him prepare the inner feeling of your physical body to touch.

Pour lips on his empty body, hug him with kisses; his face, his chickens and stomach, and the smooth cock. A drop of hot air on your skin and hands crying to your house, back and shoulders.

Walk gradually and with each move you look at their reaction. Stand against the attack, show him the desire and pray correctly.

Increase your contact and get more excitement; the body works on the body and scratches to apply the axis and then slowly cools the pressure to an irreversible point. Repeat this process several times until the exciting pressure is released.

Take a woman to a man and show her that you care for and love her, don't use her or throw her away. Tell her she still needs more sex, even later.

Start speaking well about how clever she thought of her, and I look forward to showing you what you mean this day. Ask her about the sense of mind, have fun on board and express your gratitude for what she says. Sit down and focus your eyes on her; Keep your hand on the walk and keep on sight. Contact the skin to disrupt his heart.

Put the pillow in the present; kisses are very emotional in women, they look at them and close directly from the tongue to the lips. Let your hands push on your shoulders, raise your nipples and increase your pressure. The greater the voltage, the greater the voltage. For many women, breastfeeding is as sensitive as a restaurant.

Proceed to the genitals; continue kissing and provoke the ugly; get a clitoral feeling with your tongue; He is very proud of many people, he feels very happy. Make it good and as long as possible. Oral sex sets orgasm higher than usual.Overall, there is no real time set for this activity; if you can both control the heat and know that the peak will come right after that.

## USE THESE POWERFUL TIPS TO ENHANCE YOUR LOVE WITH SKILLS

One of the challenges for married and long-term couples is how to burn a fire. Sometimes the problem with the couple is too comfortable that their life is already losing spunk. On the other hand, there are couples who have the problem of losing the love or tension they feel about each other. What should you do if this is the case?

In short, you need to learn how to improve your love life or improve your love relationship - which also means learning how to improve your love abilities.

How To Improve Love: A Fragrant Thing!

So the first step you need to take to improve your love relationship is to light the bed. While it is true that relationships should not be based solely on sex, it plays an important role when you join as a couple.

We say that you always do deeds within the limits of your bedroom. Giving sex outside the bedroom is a sure way to stimulate things and improve your love. No doubt the new environment will contribute to the action - whether you are doing it in the kitchen, living room or wherever there is no bed. The excitement of a fast pigeon or even the whole session increases with love for love.

Another thing to keep in mind to improve your love is to stay out of your comfort zone. Even the very act of asking for a new position in bed, using sex toys or playing roles will fill the fire in your sex life so you can improve your love relationship at the same time.

Most men forget to bring love back into a relationship - this is something you need to be aware of if you are willing to work to refine your love techniques and save your relationship. . Or have you forgotten to submit to long-term failure? If you are always busy going to the main event, it wouldn't help your efforts to improve your love life. Overall, heating things in bed is not the best thing to try new things and adapt to the needs of your family.

For most couples, personal love plays a very important role in bed and is more important than anything else if you want a strong relationship with each other. Feel free to try new things and return your old days!When you think about it, the preliminary program involves contacting, contacting the mayor or hands, or even meeting your breath for your loving person.If we can improve the quality of contact, more predictable sexual energy is created.

Simple predictive exercises

The best way to contact our partner is to do a simple exercise. This is the best way in your body to learn a new skill than to think about it.

And yes, thinking about sex is the worst thing you can do. Most women are very sensitive to energy and attention to humans. It feels very much if you just want to give your head, not sexual energy and pleasure.

The exercise is to give someone you have a passion for expressing ideas for a minute. Change it now and contact your feelings, joy and feelings.

Ask your love love what best contact you made. You will find that the more you are present in your fingers and the less you are in your head, the more joy your partner will get.

More tips for predicting

- Take your time
- Contact slowly
- Contact every part of the body, including the inner legs, toes, hair and toe
- Take time to romance with the breasts
- Use your lips and tongue
- Blow your beloved body
- Use fur, silk and feathers

Speak dirty to increase sexual energy (see below)

Take the projected experience and the emotions of sex.

Now you can extend these tips with sexual intercourse. The more attention you have to pay for penis feelings, the more energy is transferred to someone you love and the more motivated it is.

For the best use of your sex life, it is important that you work smoothly in preparing your predecessor. We hope to look at some common prediction tips and highlight what you shouldn't do, and we can increase your sexual ability and improve sex.

A prediction is a set of physical or psychological activities designed to stimulate sexual stimulation or motivation. While the most obvious techniques such as touch and kiss come at first glance, other actions, such as speaking or even a text message, can be viewed as an introduction.

In women, foreplay is absolutely necessary at the physiological level, because foreplay is responsible for increasing and lubricating the vagina, which means that sex can penetrate without pain.

Women usually like to make pines, so they feel they are more rated than sex, so all activities must be done with patience and sensitivity. Small dirty speech is suitable for heating. You can tell a woman exactly what you want to do and slowly begin to imagine sexual action, which makes her excited. Women want to be respected and open up their trust and trust in sexual conversation with them.

For the best use of your sex life, it is important that you work freely when preparing for your predecessor. We hope to go through some forecasting tips and highlight what should not be done, and we can improve your sexual ability and improve your sex.

A predictor is a series of physical or psychological activities designed to encourage sexual stimulation or motivation. Although the most visible techniques such as contact and kiss are seen at a glance, other actions, such as speech or even a text message, can be considered as an introduction.

In women, forging is absolutely necessary at the physiological level, because forging is responsible for increasing vagina and lubricants, which means that sex can penetrate without pain.

Women usually make pine trees, so they feel more valuable than sex, so all activities must be done with patience and sensitivity. A small, dirty speech is suitable for warming up. You can tell a woman exactly what you want to do and start thinking about sexual behavior slowly, which makes her excited. Women want to be respected and open up their trust in sexual conversation with them.

Some men never seem to understand. Women are not battery-powered toys and can be turned on and rolled up for fun at any time - despite the appeal of this image to many men. If you are like most men, it is certain that you will give the woman you are in a state of sexual delirium. You've probably spent some time studying various sexual techniques that claim you can do it sexually, and you've probably tried several. You've probably found out what other men have found: sex is more than just tricks and techniques. The secret of better sex is its beginning than even foreplay. Here are some better tips for predicting sex to be crazy!

The first is simple: start with his mind. In most women, sex in the brain actually begins and usually before sexual intercourse.

For this reason, you can plant the seeds for intimacy at the beginning of the day using gentle smoothness, hugs and soft kisses on the next and on the neck. When it comes to better tips for sexual whitening, it's invaluable! You'll be surprised how a bit of litter in the morning after all day thinking and allowing her to increase her desire can lead to a lot of fun in the morning.

If you see it later in the day, pay attention but don't overflow it. The goal is always to remind her that she is as desirable as you are and to establish a personal relationship later in the evening. Better tips for sexual predictions often include things that are forgotten as tricks and a thin touch. You don't want to move her legs, but you'd better touch her gently, which is wise and expect signs of sexual contact.

The improved sexual prediction may also include verbal communication. Whisper here and there - tell her what you want to do with her and let her ideas encourage the images of passion she faces. The key is to allow her brain to work on each cylinder so that its prospect is shot to the boiling point.

Remember - it's all about the brain, and everything in your foreplay is designed so that his brain wants as much as it loses perspective when it's time for sex. There are better tips for sexual predictions that include actions such as teasing feet or leg feet - a game called "Footsie". Remember, many of the old techniques are still among the best!

And when it's time to get to the last level, don't jump into the game immediately. These challenges must continue until sexual intercourse begins. Kissing, caressing, licking and squashing her body to strengthen her desire to be at the height of her sexual desire when sexual intercourse begins. If you can be patient enough to use these better sexual prediction tips, you will be sexually crazy to remember days and weeks.

If you spend a lot of time on high quality foreplay, you can bring your wife pleasure to new heights of ecstasy. Prediction is an essential part of helping your wife gain severe orgasms.

To get the most out of your preliminary work, think more than just how to iron and care for a woman. It's not just about physical stimulation. Instead, it inspired your wife's mind.

By encouraging her mind, open the door to help her not only find simpler orgasms, but also facilitate easier orgasms. Adding diversity is a good way to energize your partner's mind during the introduction.

An example is the use of a variety to get something different into the bedroom every day. This is not necessarily a physical instrument. Instead, introducing something as simple as you change with your wife can be very difficult if you do it right. Another example could be changing the way you make love. In other words, if you are a species that uses a very gentle approach, you may find that erotic fantasies for a partner can cause the partner erotic emotions that can be enhanced. .

However, it is important to note that you must first understand the possibilities and want a general gender for women before you can make any sudden changes. The last thing you need is that things are very productive. The only way to add any kind of diversity to your bedroom is to maintain a high level of respect, trust and communication between you and your partner.

By taking the time to use these powerful mental stimuli during foreplay, you can help your partner be so overwhelmed that when he finally reaches his orgasm, he becomes the new peak.

## BREATHING TECHNIQUES TO IMPROVE SEXUAL PERFORMANCE

We all know that it can hinder the transformation "too fast" when we are with our other half. Whether we've met or someone we've had for a long time, we want to join and enjoy as much as possible. Many conditions can be destroyed by a lack of sexual engineering in the bedroom, but don't worry ... help is available!

When we are at the moment, it is very difficult to realize that we have to do something as simple as stopping and breathing. It has been shown that this technique can significantly limit you and bring you back to your surroundings. The most common reason for premature winding up for sex is too early! The best way to ensure that this does not happen is by breathing regularly. If you notice your breathing, you will probably survive much longer than normal.

The best way to do this is ... If you think you're too excited, take a deep breath and slow down your speed. Then make sure you take a breath and continue at a regular pace. Remember, this is a marathon, not a sprint!

Finally, when you reach the top, it is proven that your breath can keep your orgasm back! So when you're going to get an orgasm, take a deep breath and keep it. You will find that there is more sensitivity and a much better experience than you are if you simply let go.

## Why you should learn different sex techniques and positions

How boring would it be to wear the same clothes every day? Or eat the same food every day? The same goes for sex. Most men and women feel that their sex life is stuck in a corner, but then they do little about it. Indeed, if these people had to spend some time learning new sexual techniques and positions and then applying them to their sexual lifestyle, they will definitely find that there is much more of their lives than they were given.

Most people try the mission when they have sex that is considered to be the most natural sexual situation. The missionary is what people use even though they have never seen anyone else. But while the missionary might be in good condition, would it not be too boring to use it every night?

Fortunately, there are various sexual techniques and positions that can be used quite effectively. Just the various options are available on the Internet itself. You will find different positions, even some videos, and you will probably have to use a lot of them. What do you stop there?

Sex is about being different. You are different than you normally are. That's part of the excitement of it all. But if you have a single partner and they see you doing the same thing with them every time, they might be looking for some variation. Yes, it is good to say that learning sex techniques and positions can save marriages and bring partners closer because this is a particularly secret connection they share with each other.

So do not undermine the power of sexual techniques and positions. Learning about them is as important as learning different recipes for preparing different meals each day and shopping for more clothes to look different each day.

If you ever want to give your partner the best sex, you should definitely learn the best sex work. This information is better than any other lover. In this section I will tell you exactly what you need to do to become the best ...


Men make many mistakes in sex that even destroy the best sex work. The first part of this book is to make sure you don't make these mistakes, because doing so will destroy the best sexual posts. Women are understood as sexual and sexual love. With that in mind, I will tell you the mistakes men make, the way to correct them, and the best sexual situation.

The best mistakes boys make during intercourse:

Looking at sex positions in porn

It's a bad idea to take sex work from porn, because the stars don't use the best sex settings, but the ones that look best on the camera. Some of them are very bad for sexual pleasure. The question of her favorite sex work is a good start

Let her do everything that works when she is on top:

Women sometimes want to be in control, but don't let them get tired before u take charge again . Do some work

Women love sex and like to crush and attract (at the height of sexual pleasure). Read it again. If you have a romantic kiss as a guide, you will immediately push it, then you will notice that it is not sexy. If you have sexual tension, it will eventually be hard and fast - after love!

Then make sure you tell her that what is happening at the height of sexual pleasure simply plays a role by kissing her and telling her that you feel very close to her and that she is a beautiful woman.

Can't last long enough to satisfy her:

Again, if I told you the best positions for sex, it would be wasted on a man suffering from premature ejaculation. Like impotence, this is very easy to cure and I will reveal how I did it!

The culmination is the whole point behind any sexual contact in which a woman or man is involved, because when a man or woman reaches orgasm, an indelible, pleasant feeling that is not comparable can be suppressed. Fortunately, it is no problem for men to achieve this wonderful feeling; however, this is not true for most women.

If a woman wants to get into the bedroom with such pleasure, she must take certain measures leading to orgasm, especially if she wants to achieve more. Of course, an important part of anticipating helping a woman is pleasure and orgasm without getting into the vagina. However, if a woman wants to peak during vaginal penetration, she must try some sexual work. The following is a description of the five most enjoyable sex positions for women, who are very popular with women.

## BEST SEX POSITION TO LEARN TO MAKE HER SCREAM LOUD

### First position -Missionary

Most women have to experience a pernicious orgasm during sexual intercourse, often having to enter deeply. And when it comes to deep penetration, nothing interferes with the missionary sex situation where a woman lies on her back when a man reaches the top. If you want to add another component of the female pleasure factor, her partner can use her fingers to stimulate the clitoris.

## Second Position - Change your mission

As in the case of a traditional mission, in the case of a change of mission for men, it is ensured that the man goes deep into the woman and lets the staff shake and inspire her clit while pushing. To remove this position, a woman puts one of her legs over her partner's shoulder to knock the angled side.

## Third Position - Doggy Style

The sexual position of the dog is very effective because it helps every woman to have fun, and we hope that the orgasm will become obsolete during sexual intercourse.

The only thing a couple should do for this sexual position is to hand over the woman at 90 degrees or go to her hands and knees and bend her. The man then goes into the vagina from behind. While the man seems to have full control, the woman can take control of the speed and power of her partner's lights.

## Fourth position - Cowgirl

This sexual situation can bring a woman the joy of her unprecedented joy if done right. Cowgirl's position allows a woman to sit on top of a man and accept her partner's place and do the work.

## Fifth Place - Changed Doggy Style

The last position in this section implies that the woman on her stomach completely flat. Then her partner places the pan so that it sits just above her pelvis. This allows the bodies to touch their G spot, and one is still able to reach the clitoris for further stimulation.

Everyone is surprised at what sexual positions are the best sex ever. We would like to satisfy all our partners if we love them. So, to get the best sex of all time, it's important that you try to create sex sites that are fun and exciting for sexual entertainment.

Society has the misconception that men should get into women as a jackhammer and that women are happy to stop. This is often done in romantic movies, but in real life it rarely happens.

The problem with film problems is that sex begins and ends when a man arrives. This is usually considered a result of love. The problem is that she completely ignores women who reach orgasm during sexual intercourse. The truth is that men come quickly and women rarely come. Don't think it's a threat to your identity. This means that you should not treat the sex as to whether you come or not, but you can. Sometimes the difference is as simple as using different types of stimuli. For example, it is important to encourage a woman to fasten her fingers and bodh during pine and sex. This gives her a long-term experience and warms up to gain orgasm first. Unlike men, the mood of women becomes gradually and is built with hope. Thus, this stimulus will not only be considered as an accidental incident, but as something that can prolong sex and lead to further orgasm.

If the girl doesn't come yet, you can try something else. For example, if you want a woman to come in during vaginal intercourse, try a new sexual condition. This has very practical advantages.

Different sites support it in different ways. Just sitting or convincing her can make a big change to get the effect. Diversification into different positions increases diversity, which can still be exciting. Some positions help to live longer with sex to gain more orgasms and become shy.

Here are some sex positions for the best sex ever. For best results, I strongly recommend warming up first by encouraging your finger to be thrilled.

This alone will create more orgasms and rise sharply as it reaches its peak. Moisten your fingers and enter and place your fingers. Then slowly slow down. Spread another finger over her clit and lick it with your tongue. She will be very concerned about this encouragement. When you get into it, you tried with the woman upstairs. This allows it to move at its own pace and adjust the angle and depth of penetration. Another advantage is that it provides a clitoral stimulus that is likely to stimulate it. He often likes slow sex, but as often as he loves to come hard. I would like to add a warning word to both posts. I strongly recommend that her hips be held in case she is too excited, which can have painful consequences.

After trying these sexual work, try to get into it while tearing it apart. This can be very exciting. You can achieve orgasm even if you're right. One of the other key features of this gender environment is that the deterioration shows that there are many leaders who psychologically attract many women. I would like to come up with your own changes. When you are in the shower, you can try some useful things and krannóg like shower!

Finally, I would like to say that each of these gender settings can be changed in different ways. For example, if you look into their eyes and do one of these things, love becomes more intense. Her weapons in a missionary state sometimes show sovereignty that she can encourage. It slows down your movements and allows it to detect each piston, greatly contributing to a sensible romantic desire you may be unlike other faster strokes. By adding these new moves and variations you will see that they reach orgasms more often than you have ever seen.

There are several exciting sexual tasks that are known to improve orgasms especially for both sexes. During sexual intercourse it all comes into place.

Did you know that setting a centimeter variation can change the orgasm feeling completely changed and the intensity level of the top line? Therefore, it is important to try the bedroom with the angles used in each location to get the best not only for yourself but also for your partner.

**Sexual position to improve women's orgasm**
A teaching mission, also known as a cow, is one of the simplest and most effective sexual tasks a woman can achieve orgasm. This position is

comparable to the known missionary position, but the only difference is that the woman is upstairs rather than the man. In a receding mission, the woman has full control over the speed and force of friction on her clit and in her place.

In most cases, it is advantageous for a woman to reach a peak in front of men. When a woman feels almost having an orgasm, she and her partner can change their position to give men more control. As you change your legs, not completely change your sexual contact, it can help you change it by separating yourself or getting closer - working on yourself. for me.

**Sexual position to improve male orgasm**
While many men consider missionary work as a reward, you prefer not only to give a dog's sexual position not only by providing excellent control, but also by providing other unpredictable benefits. For example, if he has sexual intercourse with this position, the man who meets the partner is likely to increase. During sexual intercourse, men can reach other erogenous belts such as back, neck, clitoris and breasts.

Of course, for all the above advantages, penetration control is the best. During a dog's sexual situation, a man can enter a woman as deeply as he wants, which brings great pleasure and joy to both sides. However, make sure it does not touch its cervix, as this can cause a lot of pain.

As you continue the experiment in the bedroom with new and exciting sexual sites, you will soon find that many of them are very similar. And after a while there is a good chance that the positions you like will be the most boring and boring. That is why you must not only discover new sex positions, but also create tension in your sexual contact.

In short, it hurts to fight sex with your partner in an interesting and resourceful way - getting sex somewhere else or an unusual part of your home, or maybe integrating food or sex toys into your sex.

Most men face a common challenge in deciding on the best sex positions when they are in bed with their girls. Most of them are not afraid, but their girlfriend would be bored if they repeat the same sexual position each time they love. Always remember that the same age always produces boring fruit. So it's usually surprising what are the best sex positions when they love?

So one of the best ways is to explain what you shouldn't do while doing sex. Most people try to imitate the sites they see in some porn movies. This is one of the main reasons most men fail when they have sex. Most men do not experience the need to watch porn movies before having sex with their girl.

I think porn is best when they see some of the best sexy hitting tablets ... That's something they can be told! Always remember that porn movies use sex pages so viewers can see and enjoy them. This is definitely not the best position for you!

You have to realize that one of the worst tasks is when women put their ankles on their shoulders because they feel pain during sex. This is one of the best positions that can be associated with all satisfaction in your sex life. The second point to keep in mind is that you are not trying to keep your weight away from your girlfriend. Certainly women can be closer to her husband. So if you continue to do your best work, you may want to be with you.

So try to gain weight the next time sex can detect it. When they have sex, most women suffer when they feel the weight of her husband on her body. Try to gain weight to say that she is able to get dirty after having sex. Avoid sharpening to keep their pub for a long time, as it can hurt.

Always remember that if your women are above them, you should not let her do her position. Sex is generally considered a passive act for most women. So if you work less, you may lose all interest with you. Don't destroy the whole purpose of having sex with your girlfriend. If you both have the same interest, you can keep one of the best sex sites.

Most men try to read books and think they are from March before sex. You must try to be an alpha hand before you get sex. The best positions are when you move your girlfriend and she turns around and you are a little aggressive. Treat her like a doll and try to change position when you have sex.

If you're reading a book on sex education, you're likely to get lots of positions, including missionaries, dog-style, 69, etc.

I think these sexual works will lose all the ship because they forget everything that even allows women orgasm, and that it is clitoral stimulation.

The problem with all sex positions is that they all rely on vaginal stimulation to bring a woman to orgasm. However, vaginal stimulation is the least effective way to induce a woman to orgasm.

In fact, there are two types of female orgasms.

Clitoral orgasm occurs when stimulating the clitoris. And then there is a vaginal orgasm that occurs when the vagina is immediately stimulated.Most sexual guidelines focus on vaginal stimulation, but few even talk about stimulating the clitoris!

Some experts do not understand that both orgasms depend on the clitoris. So it is not the logical art of clitoral motivation to dominate.By reading this book, you can become a very powerful lover and turn a woman into an orgasm using the technique I am going to share with you in every sexual work.

So what is the technique that improves the sexual situation? What the hell! Now I'm not good, just using the right term! You need to grind her very well.

How to use this sexual technique: Take every sex position and focus on penetrating. Turn your dick into a sex action! When entering your partner, turn the body clockwise. Clitoral pressure and stimulation, which can lead to an explosive female orgasm.

Then try again if you love your partner. Take any sexual position and add a screw movement to it. You would turn average sexual techniques into powerful orgasm producers.

Start with a simple thing like a mission. Simple work as an anti-mission gives you the opportunity and time you use this simple method to attract a woman to dominate.That's all you need to do to do any sexual work that

has turned into a powerful female orgasm..

## FOUR REASONS WHY YOU SHOULD BRING SOME NICE SEX POSITIONS IN YOUR SEX LIFE

A close relationship is an essential element of any long-term romantic relationship. A common factor to be separated is that partners do not maintain their sexual relationship. There is something that can keep the soul and body. To keep the sexual aspect of your relationship active at all times, consider testing fun sites sometimes. Here are 4 reasons.

1. sex position spice up a relationship. It's a very good medicine, it's a pleasure to add to the sex monotony of a relationship. And what better way to add sex than to try a creative and new position? You see that if you do the same things over and over again, sex becomes routine. When sex is routine, it's easy to get bored of describing you. If you allow your sex to not happen, change your relationship. Satisfaction with sex is a solution that can stop depression and promote a close relationship in your relationship.

2. It can highlight your climax. If you want to do this for yourself or your partner to get an orgasm and be difficult in normal sexual contact, try some new sex fun positions. These positions are helpful to your partner, especially when it comes to women, to end and have an incredible orgasm. This site is important to bring happiness to your partner.

Editing part of your basic tasks can really start the fun. By accurately focusing on the site through the right websites, you and your partner can expect you to have the most unusual sex ever.

3. It can reduce your stress. Going into a sexual routine can create a stressful relationship. It would not be good if you or your friend had sex if you had a duty. It turns into another story about humorous sexual posts. By breaking the

famine, these types of positions can bring joy and happiness into contact.

If you look forward to something that brings you so much pleasure, you can help your body produce hormones and release them, which can reduce stress levels. If you want to ease the tension in your relationship and rehabilitate the herb, try to move away from your normal sexual situations and try fresh and unknown.

4. Live much longer. For these three reasons, it helps you and your partner spend a longer life looking for fun positions. Statistics show that sex itself has the potential to improve your body's natural protection against diseases and disorders. Add to this the benefits you can gain from joy and laughter, such as medicine and slowing down the aging process.

These are good reasons to see sex from a different perspective. In this way, you can open yourself to several features that can give you and your partner more pleasure and enjoyment.

When it comes to a close sexual relationship, many women are suspicious of men they think they are taking and have little result. In many cases, sex is another "task", such as washing or washing clothes, or a negotiating chip for washing or washing. On the other hand, many men see women as sexual curiosity and treat them as such. Many are here for the "thing" that they can acquire and withdraw if they are not physically, emotionally.

And if the sexual relationship is not amazing, the unhappy partner concludes that there is not enough love in the relationship or that something is wrong with the other. Similarly, if there is a significant difference between the ideas of one partner, the needs and fantasies of one partner, one or both of them will find that something is contrary to the other - and / or relationship. Their own feelings, expectations and motivations are generally not dubious, but do not move on to another relationship.

The continuing inability to "sexual satisfaction" leads to a constant search for new sexual partners and new sexual experiences. For some people it is worth a lot of unusual sex to stay in a relationship that does not meet all other aspects.

This ongoing search for new sexual partners, new sexual experiences, new sexual techniques and new sexual outfits happens in some way as a ceremonial duty and dependence on some people. This "horny" model of sex is rather than "sex from the vacuum" than "sex from the whole". He accepts that we are "sexually fulfilled" once we reach orgasm so that we can continue and sleep.

Yes, we can achieve or raise other heights on multi-tier platforms by encouraging the other sex to make precise technical specifications or using cutting-edge technologies. But while technology is an important part of love and for some sexual devices, the body jumped to reach orgasm, although an off-road close relationship takes us from what is really going on.

The outer part (the body) is the only part of us that we would like to "expose" others. The inner part is another story. We cannot encourage him to share it as a theater of jealousy, anger, long-term anger, emotional wounds, memories of painful humiliation, confusion, fear of inadequacy and rejection, false expression, discipline and conflict, doubt, confusion and shame.

It's easy to get used to physical sex and have the most vulnerable aspect of our God (inner self) because when we are inside we are the most vulnerable. In an effort to protect us, the brain brings out all sorts of excuses, reasons, and alternatives that allow us to discover our inner vulnerability. Because our brain understands vulnerability only negatively, we have no reference to how we can consciously abandon or release our normal sexual boundaries, fear, fear, shame.

When released, he is often young, rebellious, blind, ruthless and dangerous. If we are ashamed or injured at these times, it only reinforces our concerns about sex and sexual relations.

We have more sexual relationships about what is inside us than about the type of body we have, the techniques we know, or the gadgets we use. The point is to be honest, honest and personal to our sexual self and to have a healthy concept and relationship to our sexual law.

We must accept and demand who will experience a close sexual relationship in order to be aware of sexual compliance; our own minds, our own bodies, our own emotions, our own lives and our own sexual bed. We must stop presenting ourselves as we wish to see us, and not reveal ourselves to any other goal, but to be "known" in a personal, valuable and personal way.

This often means that we have to eliminate almost everything we have ever learned about sex in the library and recipes, and throw away draft reports of what works: touch your ear and rub for four minutes, neck kiss for two minutes, another finger back in small minutes another two minutes, soft to the left and directly climb your feet 90 degrees, counting up to fourteen - and all sorts of mechanical friction.

We must try to know what works for us as dynamic and versatile people and as a couple with hearts, emotions and the ability to experience the unknown and the unconscious.

We must be vigilant, open, self-confident and cheap to observe the intuitive and spontaneous erotic consequences of our hearts and souls, not the waste of our brains or "sexual experts".

Only by entering this door to inner vulnerability and surrender without help are we truly intimate sexual. Intimacy itself is a self-reflective process rooted in the concept of surrender - our own elements that cannot be controlled, energetic, spontaneous, incredible, uncertain and closer to the main natural forces. We are surprised at what we experience in these new openings and changes. The intensity of our erotic desires, emotions, desires and impulses and the level of awareness of what we do at the time we do is more important and more vital than all bedroom maneuvers, techniques, and tactile tricks.

When we decide whether we are sexually happy, the most vulnerable, the most unmanned, we overcome most of our own, shouting "Oh my God" between orgasm.

This is a close sexual relationship from intoxication. There is a great feeling that he is finally "known"; an intense, energetic and exciting experience of having a sexual connection with another person.


But to come here, we need to be fully aware and present at the moment. We cannot worry whether we will be an orgasm or not, because we will not fully accept the experience; we and our beauty partner will steal sexual relationships.

When we are very enthusiastic about sexual activity, we have noticed that there is a strange noise, everyday reality continues and our life ends on the edge of our bed. We continue until our minds, our emotions, our minds and our minds, not just our body,!

When we are willing to affirm ourselves - spirit, emotion, body, soul and spirit - the bedroom becomes a place where the sexual self can fully manifest and the spiritual self celebrate two spirits, two bodies, two. soul and two ghosts. It is usually called sexual ecstasy or sexual cross.

Sometimes sexual techniques, sexual aids or even sexy clothes are undesirable because wisdom is the soul and the generosity of the mind of much higher quality.

When it comes to sexual intimacy with deep intensity and ecstatic depth, most of us are still virgins. We may have had sex or loved and had several orgasms with one or more partners, but many of us still have to "DO" or let "DO" - mind, emotions, body, soul and spirit.

There is no intention that poor sexual performance leads to many problems in relationships and marriages. This is a fractional fact and the importance of gender in any relationship. Little is available from persistent sex tips in the modern world that help men stay in bed longer. He did nothing to increase the occurrence of couples' orgasms and did not help people be happy.

The tantric principles of sexuality are the basis of all sexual success and satisfaction. Not only do they leave men longer in bed and have better sexual performance in the bedroom, they are also great for enhancing the relationship with the bedroom. Here is information about this policy.

Powerful sexuality techniques are not new tantra throughout the world, and it is surprising that there are very few people. Because fewer people use these techniques in their everyday lives, people during sexual intercourse maximize their emotional satisfaction and sensory outbursts. These are the tantric principles of sexuality that help people achieve. When implemented correctly, these policies are great, so couples can not only develop skills to increase growing orgasm, but also have long-term orgasms as often as they want. with them.

Studies have always shown that it is easy to stay longer in bed and work well in the bedroom. This is what every woman wants, and the only known acronym for better sexual satisfaction. However, modern lifestyles emphasized immediate satisfaction, so everything people look for is instant entertainment and creates shortcuts in life. While this may be good for some aspects of our lives, it does not help people enjoy more sex. Not only is it a major cause of premature ejaculation and other malfunctioning genitalia, but it is also the real sex of her joy and relationship.

Tantra sexual techniques emphasize increased sexual stimulation through a spiritual approach to sex and satisfaction. By allowing couples to connect their bodies and minds, the couple can push the boundaries of pleasure and sexual satisfaction in the bedroom. As techniques adopt a spiritual and mental approach to sexual intercourse, they usually improve a person's peace of mind during sex, allowing them to better control their level of tension. Therefore, a man can prevent premature ejaculation and stay in bed longer

Statistics show that the number of women suffering from orgasms during intercourse. Not surprisingly, most people in the world do not have satisfactory relationships, especially given the importance of sex in sexual relationships. The problem is usually how men and women deal with sexual intercourse in the bedroom. Thanks to tantric sex tips, all couples can re-learn their approach to sex, and thus learn to increase the intensity of pleasure during sexual intercourse.

Instead of focusing on instant sexual satisfaction, like most couples, Tantric sex techniques have focused on extending sexual stimulation and increasing intimacy. With today's satisfaction of the world with immediate satisfaction, it is not surprising that many people suffer from premature ejaculation. This means that most men cannot stay in bed for a long time and therefore cannot satisfy their partners.

Tantra sexual tips usually emphasize couples who need time during sexual intercourse because they need a more spiritual approach to sex and love. With the slow growth of stable sexual energy in the bedroom, orgasms usually spread, which usually last longer than most spouses in the modern world.

A common problem in today's world is the failure error. This is usually due to unrealistic expectations about sex. Usually this is due to misconceptions because people view sex as a short session to continue with sexual desire. This usually causes a lot of stress because people are concerned about what their partners think about their performance. There is no problem with tips on tantric sex.

Tantric philosophy is very different because it requires a different sexual approach. It puts more emphasis on being calm and more focused on the heart and mind than on the frequency of functions and penetration. Sexual tips based on this philosophy are therefore good to help one stay at peace with himself and his partner, allowing him to stay longer in bed.

Personal bans are one of the main causes of lack of sexual satisfaction and orgasms in modern relationships. People are usually brought up with a misunderstanding of sex and some believe that sex is necessary, but others believe it is only for physical satisfaction. This usually clarifies their spiritual nature and therefore leads to lower levels of relationships. Tantra sexual techniques have a different approach where couples learn to respect sex as a great gift of nature and pleasure.

With the right attitude to sex there are usually better orgasms involving couples who use tantric sex tips and encounter sexual intercourse. Men can usually stay in bed with these techniques to get full sexual pleasure.

## INCREASE SEXUAL ENDURANCE - 4 SIMPLE TIPS FOR INCREASING SEXUAL STAMINA

Most men can only spend a few minutes having sex. It may be due to embarrassment and frustration that you have a low level of sexual endurance. It also delayed me and I did some research and learned how to stay in bed longer.

Follow these tips and learn how you and your wife can enjoy the best sex you have ever had.

### 1. Eat improved sexual stamina

Design your diet on foods that are known to increase sexual stamina. Mild blueberry is in my opinion a good food to increase sexual stamina. It contains vitamins and minerals that improve sexual stability better than any pill or drink. Stay with natural foods such as fruits and vegetables and try to avoid all fast food. Regular use of a healthy diet improves sexual performance and bed stability.

## 2. See how you breathe during sex

Body tension kills long-term sex, so watch out for how to feel in bed. This tension increases the chances of premature ejaculation and other problems. Breathe deeply and slowly and focus on your breathing patterns.

Try to do it naturally, not a mandatory rhythm. You can breathe your partner for a more combined feeling.

## 3. The secret sexual technique always works

If you want to stay in bed tonight, try this technique. This will increase your sexual stamina and give your wife a good time. Start inserting your penis as far as possible. Make sure it's comfortable for your wife. The trick is to leave it without ironing and move your hips only in a circular assembly. It works because one is the most sensitive part of the body and it gets inside the vagina more and more. So if you stay deep inside, there will be less friction and you will have better control of your ejaculation. This position provides excellent inspiration for the clit that women love.

## 4. PC Cone Muscle Workout

You can prepare at any time to improve your sexual stamina using cone exercises. They are easy to execute and work on PC muscles that control your ejaculation formation. Simply hide the muscles as if it was flowing through the urine to do it. Change the number and maintain time for bends to see good results quickly.

Remember, these tips are just the first step to increasing sexual stamina. For the long-term control of the ejaculation you want ... more help is needed.

It's a great start to building sexual stamina with these ideas, but expect a complete course of different exercises to help you permanently increase sexual stamina.

Orgasms, if properly raised, can experience a great sexual experience. All you need is good practice and knowledge of explosive bachelor's techniques. In fact, the whole process of sexual relationships is not just a combination of motivations and reactions. You create a number of stimuli in your wife's body, leading to a series of related reactions that lead to mutual enjoyment.

There are places in women's bodies that can be fools when they are excited. These places are the best place for bumpy orgasms. Depending on the sensitivity of this site, a faster orgasm will lead to some of them and lead to a slow orgasm to others. Of all the sexually sensitive areas of the female body, G is considered the best place to give her a quick orgasm.

Position G can be easily placed in the vagina. You can distinguish between a slightly rough structure compared to the inside of the vaginal walls. In addition, it is somewhat dark compared to the pink color of the vagina.

Try watching with your finger. It is located in front of the vagina and is near the front wall.

Everyone is disappointed with sex. But few people try to make a love session great, full of joy in life and never before pleasure. If you want to give your wife and yourself elegant sexual pleasure, use sexual techniques that are always aimed at hitting the G-spot.

Leave it loops on your knees like a dog with its back to you. Then go to his sexual recession. Ask her to spread her legs as much as possible. Then insert it with a pencil and push it down towards the main wall of the vagina. Do not use fast movements. Walk slowly with proper friction movement and hit point G several times.

If you are unsure about the location of G, you can use this technique: Place it in the normal bed position and go to her sexual device. After proper lubrication, you can enter not only half the body.

Then begin to move clockwise and counterclockwise near the vaginal opening. Encourage her to regularly seek out and reach an explosive orgasm in no time. Go for unlimited orgasm with this trick. The speed of the sliding force behind this position is.

There are many ways a person can improve their performance in a bedroom. Staying in bed longer is one of the easiest ways to do this. This is because the only way you can ensure that your partner continues to stimulate the vagina. If you stay in bed for a long time, you can increase your chances of getting in touch with her "G-spot" and increase her chances of getting an orgasm. This way you can stay in bed longer for better sexual performance.

The easiest way to prevent early electronic publishing is to control the intensity of your excitement. This is the only way you can take control of the ejaculation process, which plays an important role in determining how well you can postpone ejaculation. Although premature ejaculation can be stopped using common sexual techniques, such as squeezing and stopping and lowering techniques, it can take longer to try different sexual settings in the bedroom.

The "best woman" of the sexual contribution is effective in preventing premature ejaculation and long sleep. If this position is taken during sex, it will help you stay in bed longer because it is calm for you. With reduced strain on the hands and feet, ejaculation can be effectively delayed. You will also not be under pressure to give it, because it regulates the frequency of shocks and depth of penetration. Without pushing it, you will be calm. You will not be afraid that you will fail, so it will be easier for you to prevent premature ejaculation. That doesn't mean it won't be comfortable for you. This is because you can better see your breasts and the whole figure and you have sex. You will have a better angle to touch his clitoris and hips, increasing the chance of orgasm.

The sex side of 'female bikes' is almost the same as the sex side above and one that you can also use to stay longer in bed. The difference between this position and the "woman upstairs" is that she looks forward to seeing you rather than the woman you are looking at. Like the sexual position of women above, it allows you to be calm when this process takes place. If you are calm, you can postpone ejaculation because you are more focused on controlling voltage.

Another sexual position that helps men stay in bed longer than front to back. It's almost like a back door, but in this case the woman is lying flat, not standing and blinking. It is good to postpone ejaculation because your hands and feet will have less strain. It's also great that it lasts longer because it gives you complete control over the intensity and depth of penetration. Makes it easier to use other methods to stay longer in bed.

Staying in bed longer is the only sure way to please every woman you come to sleep with. Anyone can stay in bed longer if they use appropriate strategies to stop premature ejaculation. To effectively implement these strategies, it is recommended to understand how they work to delay ejaculation. The following are effective strategies to stay longer in bed and therefore allow you to have better sexual performance.

The pressing technique is a common technique used by most men to stay longer in bed. The only thing you can postpone ejaculation is to stop punishing his punishment when he thinks he's going to replace it. It is an effective remedy for premature ejaculation because it has effects on stimulation. Because pain is punished, it usually helps to prevent involuntary contractions that are usually needed to successfully stimulate ejaculation.

The pressure at the top of your thunder therefore lowers the level of tension and thus prevents premature ejaculation. To avoid disrupting the flow of sexual stimulation, it is recommended that you usually squeeze your penis only if you are encouraging. Also, you should not exaggerate this technique, as there are situations where men clench and thus interfere with their sexual performance.

Sexual technique is a start-and-stop technique that has proven useful for men who want to stop premature ejaculation. Postponing ejaculation with this method is simple, so the reason for its popularity is for men who have problems with early exhaustion. Everything you need to do to stay in bed longer than taking a break of about 20 seconds to find time to destroy and shake again. With this method you can survive as long as you want in bed.

This is an effective method to stop premature ejaculation, because breaks usually reduce the level of stimulation, so when the schedule is corrected, ejaculation can always be free because it is not possible because you enter the voltage. Active personal events will be helpful if you use this method for a long stay in bed, as there is a risk of unpleasant moments during breaks.

Because men are, by their very nature, human in terms of sex, we see in our minds the impact that we finally have on the level of tension we have. Visualization is therefore a powerful tool for delaying ejaculation. Usually, people who suffer from premature ejaculation and want to stay longer in bed are advised to think of something other than sexual activity. This distraction is usually useful in lowering a person's stress level, thus providing more bed time.

When it comes to using dense condoms and de-sensitive tablets, the logic is almost identical to the logic. The reason people use condoms as a method to stop premature ejaculation is because it promotes less penis. This is because the man has no direct contact with the woman's vagina and therefore has a lower level of tension.

This allows you to postpone ejaculation and stay in bed longer, as it will take longer for the intensity of sexual stimulation to reach the point where ejaculation occurs. Hardened pills also reduce the ability of the penis to stimulate orgasm, thus effectively preventing premature ejaculation. However, it is not a natural method to stop premature ejaculation and is therefore not recommended as a healthy way to stay in bed.

The best way to postpone ejaculation is a sexual technique that men know and swear, but usually it is a technique that you should find out yourself. This is not a special site, but a multiple method. Not only will you reach your potential in the bedroom, but she also loves it and invites you again and again.

If you are young and inexperienced (or you are not sure that you are doing), it is very easy to lose and tense again and exert pressure until things get out of hand. This is the main reason for premature ejaculation. Our pencils are heavily stimulated as we draw in, and when we do it over and over again, it's no wonder that it ends so fast for the boy.

You don't know some facts about female anatomy. The hollow tube is not a vagina, but more than an inflatable balloon. Most of the muscles at the input and limbs are excellent. The more you go to the end, the more it opens up, the muscles relax and things aren't that strong.

You can use it to your advantage. The key is to push the most sensitive part into it through its narrow entrance, but push the ground into it and stay inside. The environment will not be more relaxed for you, but will still be able to feel it at its entrance.

You can sharpen or turn your body against it because your clit is against your pocket. This technique works very well at the top because you can control it or even prevent it from moving too much. Encourage her hips to move back and forth or out, not up and down. Don't push at all until you're ready to warm things up.

This will not solve your immediate problem and finishing more often than not is a mental and physical problem. There are a lot of tips that can help you be more accessible, but this sexual method is what you can go for. So remember, go as deep as you can and don't push. It's a great way to postpone ejaculation and help her get a better time.

You are likely to face premature ejaculation if you are, and this is a problem that many other men around the world will share with you. This can lead to embarrassment and confidence, especially if you cannot satisfy your partner's wishes. But do not worry because there are ways to prevent such a barrier to make sex and improve your stamina when you love it.

Premature ejaculation is something that can happen only once or so often. This is where the male organ takes place before or before the desire or pleasure of your partner.

Remember, however, that there is no real time limit; For some couples, orgasm may be premature if it occurs within 15 or 20 minutes after sex. But it is always best to have your partner achieve their orgasm and achieve as you normally do.

The following three tips and techniques to combat premature ejaculation and improve sexual stamina:

**Withdrawal technique** - The most common technique is to pull it out before you have an orgasm; This shows that you have to expect an upcoming orgasm. Any person can anticipate their orgasm and by that time they should stop their immediate stimulus. At this point, the partner must cooperate and be informed and understandable. It will expire a few minutes and the erection is probably a bit bleeding - you can restore sex again. Alternatively, you can increase your stamina with frequent exercise. You can manipulate yourself to determine the point at which ejaculation occurs. Reduce the feeling when prompted to go again and masturbate.

**Sexual Techniques** - Think about non-sexual thoughts during a sexual act. Take a look at your mother's home kitchen or the upcoming football game. Think of the great entertainment you want to record again. This technique probably reduces your orgasm slightly, but it may affect its intensity, so be careful. A more practical way would be to use better and stronger protection. Use a stronger condom to reduce the sensation at the end of your pain. Latex reduces coated risks and STD sensitivity to genitals.

**Use of desensitizing creams** - Leave your penis numb with a special cream that will freeze your penis and allow you to exercise longer. Note, however, that this may affect your partner's motivation if they come into contact with their skin.

You can also explore the use of high quality male supplements to optimize sexual stamina. These recipes, which combine herbal extracts and nutrients, focus not only on erectile strength and quality, but also on libido, energy and endurance during the bedroom event.

Erectile disorder is a problem that can never be highlighted. If you include things, you have to pay the price because this problem is not a cold problem. Discuss with the help of an expert to find everything in the right direction. Look, these are the various construction modifications available. The best male enhancement pills should always be taken without much care. There is no doubt that people looking for all these features on the road are often wrong.

There are many reasons for your problem. It can be seen that psychological problems can be important construction problems. First, you have to heal from the mind to cure the various sexual problems you suffer.

There are only natural building pills on the best male pills for enhancement, so you should not rule out dirty options. Access must always be correct to get on the right track. The construction problem is not a genetic problem; This is the main cause of erectile dysfunction by frequent attacks on people who are not well aware of this system. It is well known that if you do not plan in the first step, there will be no more room. Any problem must be solved in the first step so that it does not disappear. Access must always be correct in every case to have the best possible way to meet your needs. Plan things and be prepared to enjoy the best sex life.

## 2 UNSTOPPABLE LITTLE PENIS SEX TECHNIQUES - GIVE HER PULSATING ORGASMS NO MATTER WHAT!

The penis is quite challenging when you have a small one. you should always have another start to make sure that you can give your full satisfaction to your partner. It is always good to learn new sex work, sexual techniques and tricks and methods. You certainly don't want to be a number or one bedroom, it can be very boring and boring. Here are some minor sexual techniques that you can use to address your lack:

1. Balloon Modeling - This particular method is a way to instantly increase your penis. There is no need to raise the penis in terms of conditions, but you do it more. This is done by maximizing the strength of your building and the blood covering the penis during construction.

First you need to fully encourage your member and you can use lubricants to help you achieve the maximum possible design. Place an elastic band or sharper object around the body base immediately after construction. It should be quite tight, but not painful or uncomfortable. This technique keeps your erection completely in your blood, giving you pain. Be sure to remove the tape just before ejaculation.


2. Add more items - you have often heard that these are small things. To get started, you can add certain things to your sexual technique. As in the mission environment, place pillows under her back to encourage her to connect better. If you are in a hands-free position, use your free hand to encourage other sensitive areas. Field like her nipples or clit.

There is nothing else to note that the most sensitive nerve endings in the vagina are in the opening of the vaginal canal, such as the first 2 centimeters. Instead of worrying about the deepest possible depth, use focus and attention to encourage this very sensitive area to open.

# 4 TIPS YOU NEED TO KNOW TO ELIMINATE SEXUAL ANXIETY

If you have ever had paranoid thoughts about going up for the chance to prepare for a sexual round with your wife or girlfriend, you are not alone. Millions of men around the world are sexually fearful and there may be more serious problems in the bedroom if it is not fixed quickly and appropriately.

While there is a great fear of sexual failure, there are effective ways to eliminate it without recourse to drugs and similar products that might escalate the problem rather than providing much needed relief. I'll show you how you can do that in a natural way if you look at the following tips and tips:

Identify the problem. The first step is to assume that you are suffering from sexual fear failure. Rejection will not only increase the problem, but sexual intercourse may be more difficult in the long run. Identify it as something you could easily arrange and you are on your way to making a complete recovery in no time.

Make a list of your positive qualities. It is a cause for concern that you are not giving sexual satisfaction to your wife or girlfriend for your confidence, not just inside but outside the bedroom.

Remember that you notice your positive qualities when you come between the sheets with your partner and you will notice some good changes immediately. The first positive thing to add to your list is that she is willing to have sex with you.

Enjoy the experience. Be careful not to focus too much on blocking your rhythm in bed - or if you are in danger. Instead of the catastrophic consequences of horizontal mambo failure, consider the sexual techniques you use to replace its strong orgasms. As another bonus you will last longer.Remember, you are not alone. The next time you become nervous in the middle of sexual contact, remember that there are millions of other men in the world who are also worried about sexual performance. Follow these simple tips and you are sure to do your job when you become intimate in the bedroom.

It is important that every man who wants to satisfy a woman stays long in bed. This is how you want to satisfy the best sexual technique with almost every woman you sleep. Ejaculation means postponing as long as you want her to learn as much as possible.

Triggering techniques and the pressing method used by men around the world to stay in bed longer are common methods. Here's what you need to know about them.

Initial and state-of-the-art technology is considered the best way to stay longer in bed because it is effective in preventing premature ejaculation while being easy to use. This way of postponing ejaculation works by disrupting the tension chain, thus preventing the sexual intensity that all men need to avoid. You also prefer men who try to prevent premature ejaculation, because it can always be used, and in this way anyone can delay ejaculation as they want. The benefit of different shocks is also that changing the shake rate can be great for your partner to guess and for good sexual performance.

All you need to do to effectively apply this method, to stay in bed longer than when you are stimulated, knock knocking. A stop of about twenty to fifteen minutes should be enough to eliminate the urge to ascend. At the end of the urge, the pole returns. The great thing about this technique is that you can use it as long as you want, which is a great way to stay long in bed.

Not only do you suddenly stop, because it can cause unsatisfactory intercourse. The speed of pressure will run down to the point of being a natural sexual skill. You can also choose other forecasting activities that you will do with your partner to ensure that you do not disrupt their chain of excitement.

With this method, anyone can prevent premature ejaculation without creams.The pressure method to stay longer in bed is the second method that slows ejaculation, which is natural and effective. It's an easy way to stay longer in bed and prevent premature ejaculation because you all have to tilt your body to gently push as you pull. Squeezing will help prevent involuntary contraction of the muscles responsible for ejaculation, effectively stopping premature deportation. Without practice this is a way to stay longer in bed, and you should try.

Premature ejaculation examinations and treatments have been rapid over the last 20 years. Many men who have previously suffered from this common problem find that there are now permanent solutions that they can easily use.Although some researchers believe it can affect as many as 1 in 3 men, most men are often ashamed to talk to their doctors and even seek treatment.

To stop this common problem, you must first understand the source. Although many still believe this problem is not physical and only psychological, studies have shown that there are links between premature ejaculation and erectile dysfunction. Therefore, some men who have addressed their problem have used a combination of treatments to achieve their goals.

Three main causes of premature ejaculation are -

- Anxiety

- Erectile dysfunction

- A tendency to rush through sexual encounters

What does this mean to you? If you are a man, the most appropriate solution is to consider the psychological aspect first. You often start researching the Internet or investing in a program that can teach you different sex techniques or offer counseling. For the most part, it is enough to fully cure and enhance sexual stamina.If you have tried psychotherapy and it is not enough to cure you, you may need to talk to your doctor to see if they recommend prescription medication for help or treatment.

Although this is not always the best choice because your doctor usually offers antidepressants that can have very negative side effects. Therefore, most people suffering from this problem are simply trying to choose a doctor as a last resort.

## SQUIRTING ORGASM: ADVANCED TECHNIQUES TO MAKE HER GUSH

It is possible for every woman to squirt. The problem is that most men have no idea how to give a woman orgasm ... But if you learn that a woman is trying to clean it will keep you as long as possible because you are rare. capacity. I'll tell you exactly what you need to get to the blistering orgasm to give her in this section.

Insert two fingers into their vagina. Make sure she is facing you and your fingers should be in contact with the front of the vaginal wall, not your back. You should feel a "G-spot". It's oval. When you finger her, you make a bid with your fingers as a "hit" while pressing on her G-point.

When you do this, you pull toward G to remove its seeds.

Women often say they want to urinate after sex. He feels that it is not urination, but an accumulation of orgasm that puts pressure on the bladder because they do not sacrifice. Of course, many women are afraid to meet their counterparts and do not allow "go out" when they get a feeling. You must ask them to rent. Do not grab it or feel it aware. Tell her it's the same type of fluid that sprays like semen or semen. She will be able to squirt.

Her ability to have a splashing orgasm also depends on the strength of her PC muscles. If her muscles are very weak, instead of splashing fluid, she can simply run away ... The stronger her muscles, the stronger her splash orgasm. There really is no limitation on how strong her orgasm can be. Theoretically, you could even make her "jump like Niagara Falls." But to get such orgasms, you have to master not only physcal techniques for sex, but also psychological.

Sex for a woman is 90% psychological. Take this part and you can get 10 times better giving bursting orgasms at night!

If you can feel so attracted to her that she sees you as your ultimate sexual fantasy, clear her emotional blockages of bad sexual experiences and set your mood so perfectly that she doesn't have sex with you, then sexual techniques she had ever had.

Since women are unable to produce as much sperm as men during ejaculation, it is thought that an outdated orgasm is equivalent to reaching a sexual peak. However, there are some misconceptions about broken orgasms. If you do not want many of the other men who felt bad in bed to make the same mistakes, read about the best mistakes men make when they give women orgasm.

## Mistake # 1: I don't know what a squash orgasm is

Briefly, orgasm is a spatter extension of the G site or clitoral orgasm. May occur after sexual intercourse or penetration due to intense orgasm combined with sexual escort. However, achieving this goal is difficult. If you want to be a master lover, do your homework and try to understand exactly what is happening to the woman's body when spraying orgasms.

## Mistake # 2: Thinking Orgasm tastes something you can give a woman during intercourse

The truth is that you should not go to wash orgasm during intercourse or penetration. The key to a woman being a splashing orgasm is to do that and sexually stimulate her, give her some oral love, or go to clit and G-spot orgasms.

As you already know, the vagina consists of different areas of pleasure and buttons - including the clitoris and the G-point. The most important thing for an orgasm is to encourage these two people first. This way, you can ensure that one of her multiple orgasms can be classified as a washed orgasm.

## Mistake # 3: Hurry up with your bags

If you want the woman you sleep to have an arbitrary orgasm, I don't want to get her. Again, remember that this is probably one of the most intense sexual experiences he may have during a pushing orgasm.

However, the gender structure of the female body differs from the way they take you. It's a significant difference. 20 minutes of stimulation immediately before the woman reaches orgasm, and it takes men only five minutes or less. So if you want to get stuck in this, don't push the whole process. Take time and enjoy long foreplay - you won't regret it.

Stay away from the biggest mistakes men and women make and maybe you were her greatest lover ever - which could be one of the most intense sexual experiences she never had. Now that you remember the mistakes men make in this aspect of sex, visit our site to find out exactly how to get an orgasm.

For men, he can make sure that the reason his partner is not squirting is not his fault. This way of thinking is ultimately self-damaging to men because you both have sex and none of you is more important than the other. In fact, there are many things that women can do to facilitate their orgasm, and their relationship with men is not at all.

Women who want female ejaculatory orgasms must understand some things: the psychological, physical, and positioning reasons that orgasm is not always steep by women.

**Psychological causes**

Many women tend to think of orgasms because they do not understand the orgasmic process. Ejaculation for women comes from the glass gland, the gland on the upper wall of the vagina. Just before they get involved, the feeling that they are about to urinate may spread. If you worry about peeing, many women will lose their sense of sexual surrender, leading to an orgasm of pressure. Women must be aware of this process in order to relax and gain orgasm. If they are allowed to feel the water, they will find that they have explosive ejaculation.

**The physical problems**

A common problem in women is weak pelvic floor muscles. When women try to strengthen these muscles using Kegel exercises, they notice a pleasant side effect: the strength and duration of their orgasms increase.

This is good news for women trying to get squirting orgasms, because weak pelvic floor muscles are a common reason why women can't burst orgasms.

## Position causes

Of course, there are many reasons why women cannot have squirting orgasms, but if you have tried everything else, it can be a position thing. Most women find it easier to ejaculate if their legs are open and their hips raised. That's why a pillow under her hips helps her orgasm.

## Triggering women to couples

As soon as you both start working on orgasms, this reinforces the point that sex is about both of you. This means you can both work together to make sex better for both of you. As soon as you communicate physically and emotionally, mind-expanding sex will soon become an important part of your relationship.

Orgasms tear apart some of the most powerful orgasms for women. Ejaculation and orgasms are a wonderful and rare experience for women.

Even the quickest Internet check reveals a situation where women literally broke it. In addition, it is amazing that men watch their wife crazy and leave completely satisfied.

Wouldn't it be great if you also gave one of those big orgasms? Guess what? Any man can bring one of these orgasms to any woman, there is only a question of some techniques.

While spraying clitoral orgasms is possible for women, most men believe it is more reliable and convenient to give her an ejaculatory orgasm G-spot. However, many boys have a problem with this: how do you get to G? Fortunately, it is easy to find this erogenous zone. Leave it on your back with your feet open and insert your finger. If this is not convenient, use routes, especially those that are water-soluble (make sure they are for indoor use). Now gently brush on her vagina.

The thing you are looking for is an area that feels a little different from the softer surrounding tissue. In general, G-spot feels a little closer than the skin on your fingers. To test if you have the right area, make a few slow moves and you should see the BIG answer from it

Now that you have a G position, a regular orgasm is usually given first. While some girls often have an orgasm without a "preparatory" orgasm, most people have to come up with an orgasm.

To give her a regular G-spot orgasm, gently tear it from top to bottom with a soft soft pole. When she is excited, she feels her vaginal balloon. This is your sign to speed up and she must have an orgasm.

The technique of washing orgasm is based on three things: fingers, wrist and hand. First, use your fingers to lightly describe your G. She should be much more excited at the moment. Some women may ejaculate at this point, but for the most part you need to add limb movement to increase speed and strength. Try to stretch your hand too much, but give it a natural secret. This movement is often referred to as "whip" in pornography because quick beakers make your hand like a whip. When it comes to orgasm, it is helpful for many men to tell their party to relax. This may be important because the orgasm may be too strong for her to last.

If you have performed all of the above steps correctly, be aware that moisture will be released as it appears. Usually it will only be a few times when it has a concave orgasm that increases as it gets used to orgasm. The key is to make sure she always likes it, whether she gets an orgasm or not. If she wants to have sex with you, it automatically increases the chances of her orgasm without trying.

If you want the best experience a person ever has for a bed, it's good to start her squirt orgasm (also known as female ejaculation orgasm). "Splashing" orgasm is good for women because it involves ejaculation and orgasm, as well as any other experience. While all types of orgasm are great for women, washing orgasm is a real help for most women because their friends have probably never been. As if that wasn't so much, women also believe that men who are among sex masters and orgasms in between have made you an essential part of their lives!

So why was he spraying orgasm on some women? The answer is certain that the technique for most men is very poor and that orgasm does not happen immediately, it requires several attempts. Many boys stop just before they start. Although there are advanced techniques that allow it to have a stronger orgasm in less time, this guide explains the basics and how to start spraying it if it has never been.

Depending on your sexual experience, this may be very easy or very difficult. Luckily, the difference between G-point hit and non-hit is quite obvious, you will notice that there is a big difference between her and her sexual disposition.

The easiest way to get this erogenous zone is to restore it and raise its hips slightly. You can use lubricants before you put your fingers in, as if you have the hands of a man 's fingers, it can be very sad to lose a place. At first move gently and turn it gently. At some point, you should feel an area a little closer than the meat around it. Try to extend this area gently to see if the sexual response is responding. If so, you have found the right place and only increase the motivation to give it a circulatory orgasm

To give her a complete orgasm, you would encourage hand and hand to use. Imagine trying to pull your body together and use this movement along with your finger to further encourage its G-point. Do not go to this stage, gradually increase your packing until you see how excited it is and its vagina begins making wet pulsating wet. At this point, it is important to ensure that they relax with their words or behavior, because many women believe that a sudden orgasmach feeling excessive to prevent them leaking. If you accept that it lasts a lot, it does bitten. When she is accustomed to it, the next time it is easier to have female ejaculation orgasm.

Squirting orgasm is something people thought was a myth: women certainly couldn't do what they used to be. In fact, the splashing orgasm is real and many couples like to experiment with this orgasm. Isn't it time you tried it, too?

The most important area you are looking for is a G-spot (you can give her a clitoris splashing orgasm, but usually it's best to start orgasm G-spot). This erogenous zone is located slightly in the upper vagina when lying on its back. The most important thing is that it should feel different from the surrounding tissue. It has a firmer structure. Once you find this area, run it gently at the end of the foreplay and you should get a great answer from it. Once you have found this area easily, you are ready for the second part of this guide: manual technology.

The first thing to handle are hand techniques. Unlike other types of sex, the most important thing about splashing orgasm is to know how to use your whole hand properly. First, you just want to gently iron the length of the G spot. Keep your movements flexible and use some grease at this early stage to make her feel better.

Once you wear a lot more and breathe (it is likely that you will feel a slight movement in the vagina, such as contraction or enlargement), slowly use more hand. The movement of your fingers should be comparable to the way you want someone to point forward. At first it can be a little intense for her, so go slowly and let her guide you through the breath and groan of pleasure.

As you approach orgasm, you can use your arms more and more. Although hand and fingers are most important, you can use your hands in a rocking motion to add more power to her orgasm. This movement also increases speed and gives it a much greater chance of starting.

Initially, it may seem difficult to give it one of these orgasms, but stick to it and continue to try these three techniques and you will soon find that it responds much better, enlarges the vagina or pulls along with each move. That's the way the body tells her you're doing everything right. At the beginning it may be a bit, but with practice you will quickly speed up her orgasm so hard that it will constantly fantasize about you, and let's face what could be better than her sexual fantasies.

Cumshot orgasm is often described as the ultimate orgasm because ejaculation gives great pleasure. Many couples often do not understand that they are those who defend themselves from being overweight.

Counseling in the field of consulting female orgasm for couples.

Orgasmic problems can start almost immediately because men do the wrong technique. First, many boys did not reach the right area. G-spot is not a small area that is clearly visible as a clitoris, you will have to feel in the right place. The tissue should feel slightly different in the G-spot area, so I often discover it and crush it a few times before applying lubrication, as it may be difficult to feel when the hands are covered with lubricants.

Take time too. While something like washed orgasm can be a quick orgasm, sometimes it takes a long time, so it gently dilutes it, first only your fingers, then slowly more and more hands and your hand. This step is often referred to as "hit" because it is similar to the way you communicate and shows where you are enjoying an orgasm. Look into her eyes and be sexually breathing while gently pulling. For this orgasm very helps to be really sex.

In fact, let her know that the erotic experience is an orgasm for you and she will respond.

Predicting is often as important as doing something really, and pushing orgasm is no exception. Many women notice that they are a little conscious when prompted, they seem to want to interfere with their own orgasm. This is where a tear can be very useful. By repeatedly bringing her to the point where she is about to find an orgasm, and then slowly revealing her orgasm, you will get used to this feeling and realize that she is part of her orchid. Once he understands it and brings you to orgasm, he recognizes that feeling and is much easier to have orgasm.

**Demolition of orgasms for couples.**

The real secret of these powerful orgasms makes her feel sexually, psychologically and physically. If both sides are covered, it is much easier for her to blister orgasm because she feels the power of all these techniques.

One may agree with this type of orgasm you have the greatest obstacle you have to overcome. Many women are afraid or affected by this type of orgasm and you need to be sure that you want to do this.

You must remember that you have to ejaculate. This is the biggest step to overcome and once you can do it, real fun can begin.

When you encourage her to help her achieve a terrified orgasm, you should focus on the place because this is how a woman ejaculates. Clitoris will give her some pleasure, but if you really want to be wild, you have to focus on the place. When excited, use 1-2 fingers to enter her body. You will want your fingers to move it "by moving here" because it will feel best for her. You can change things every day and then move your fingers in a circle. Just make sure you do everything you do always striking.

Clitoris can also be supported to speed things up. While you know you need to focus on the spot to spray it quickly, you can also support his clit. The easiest way to support both parts of your body is to use your hand with your fingers in it and thumb on the clit. This is the work you need to be there if you want to cool it down.

With this new awareness you will change the way your wife feels happy. She doesn't want to know what's going on with her, and it'll be crazy. Spraying orgasm is one of the best orgasms a woman can ever have, and once she has it, she dares for you to reach it again.

You want your girl to squirt and shake with joy. You want to give her an orgasm that is from this world. There are a number of things you can do to maintain the level of home fitness between you and your partner. The 4 points discussed below are a relatively simple guide to sexual relations:

1. Try new places of love. Love in the bedroom is sometimes bored and bored. You and your partner must try new placements to make it more interesting and bring new excitement to your love session. Places like kitchens, offices, cars, parks but and rest areas and great places to explore with your partner.

2. Try new sexual techniques and situations. In 90% of cases, your partner is willing to try new techniques and positions, but he is too happy to say so. To love, no matter how amazing the basic act, can be boring over the years. You don't have to represent things like a whip or something dangerous. There are many different ways your love can change.

3. Be better. Foreplay is very important during a sex session because they create the sexual expectations needed to make love. Especially women need more time than they get warm. But sometimes boring foreplay gets. Therefore, you need to improve your game by introducing new features such as games and role-playing situations.

Do not push the foreplay. A good foreplay should take at least 15 minutes and start with your clothes on.

4. Get better communication with your partner during sexual intercourse. Don't be embarrassed, ask your partner for feedback and instructions on how to please them. Good communication is the basis for a better love session with your partner. Let them lead and provide valuable feedback on how to improve your techniques, etc.

I am sure that if you apply these 4 points in your sex life, you will soon be able to bring the level of a close relationship between you and your partner to a new level.

One cannot do better than satisfy your partner in the best possible way. A woman can enjoy sex every time and at any time, but if you know the G-spot technique, you're her hero.

What exactly is G and how to get it? Position G is located in the vagina and is an area filled with strong nerve ends. When a woman is sexually drunk, she runs out of blood.

Position G is located on the outer wall (side) of the vagina and is two to three centimeters from the opening into the vagina. It's a little bumpy or you can feel the ridges when doing the G-spot technique. Your partner can tell you exactly where this place is because it wants to be sexually motivated.

Why is G-spot technology so important for sexual intercourse? About half of all women feel very excited when G is stimulated. This area is like a penis with blood and helps a woman have an excellent orgasm.

If I find it, what is the G-spot technology? The best way to get a G position is to have oral sex, and when excited, two fingers are inserted into the vagina by focusing on the G position.

Gently bless your fingers and keep your tongue on her clit. Feeling around and going down about two or three inches, feeling the distance flow of the rib's presence G. It is more pronounced when a woman wakes up.

What G-spot technology ensures its motivation? A lot has been said about this and some people say that the best technique is the style of the dog or girl upstairs. While they may work for some of them, others do not. None of these positions actually use penis anatomy when standing as far as possible.

Remember that the ascent rises and that the natural heel is outside G at the above points. However, there is a G-spot warranty technique that gives the person in contact with the G-spot every time. This technique is called Breaking the Gate Palace and comes from Chinese sex techniques.

The woman must lie on the table or bed and lift her legs to her chest. One cushion or cushion should support rear water from behind. The man stands in front of her and slowly enters her vagina.

The angle is correct and the glands rub the point against its G-point in excellent G-spot technique. No need for deep pressure and really the best shallow pressure. Most women will have an excellent orgasm with this technique.

Rotate between deep and shallow to slowly bring him to orgasm. The man must wait for the woman to get an orgasm until it is his turn to orgasm. A lack of deep thrust will be nice. This is a great G-spot technique that makes you a lover who is careful and careful with the needs of your partner.

You may be wondering why I call these forbidden sex techniques and what to do with sex rights. That's because they know you have sexual power over your imagination ... but they're known to everyone. It is still terrible for me and I cannot find any other reason for this or should these sexual techniques be avoided, or someone really does not want us to find out how we can have good sex we have.

Is this case fair for ordinary boys who usually have no idea how to have sex properly and what they really can? From now on, I will reveal some sexual clues about the country that I found in my research years in this section, and no one will be able to stop you from seeking more information and love men. and Miss. Here are some of my pure golden sex techniques for better sex:

If we could find out what everyone wanted ... Really, we could easily find it. How will we do it? Putting one or two fingers in the vagina and experimenting with various oral techniques we can think of. When we come to the right one, she tells us to connect her vagina smoothly. We must maintain a constant rhythm and pressure until it has an orgasm. You can also use this observation technique in other publishing situations - get different characters and see if she likes what you do.

It is very interesting how many people who seem to know everything about having sex do not know how deep the spot is and that stimulation is by far the easiest way to activate a vaginal orgasm. The Deep Spot is also known as Epicenter, Spot or Fornix Erogenous Front Zone (AFE). It is a smooth area about 3.5 to 4 inches deep in the vagina near the cervix. You can stimulate it with your middle finger - push it as deep as possible into its vagina along the main wall (use a lubricant and press it firmly together) until you feel a texture change.

Then the deep spot is massaged by curling your finger "here" and pressing your finger firmly against the smooth area of the vaginal main wall. Find the right speed and pressure by observing its reactions and do not back down or change until it jumps. After you teach her to have deep orgasms from her finger, you can also activate vaginal orgasms by massage her deep spot with the penis during sexual intercourse.

What is the most sensitive erogenous female zone? Yes, that's the brain. Many men have no idea how powerful a woman's mind is. He arranges everything. You can literally teach her how to get out of your voice without physical stimulation. If you don't let her feel the right way, nothing works.

And I don't mean anything, not even the best sex techniques in the world. A woman should feel good with you, trust you, yearn for you and above all respect you. You need to be self-confident and reliable. You must lead her. Don't tilt. You must be a man.

Why not try it - tell your wife / girlfriend when you go home that you want to make sure you don't have sex tonight. The rule doesn't matter what happens, you can't have sex. Then she teases her all night and let her wish her a lot, but don't let her have you.

When you see that she is ready, blindfolded and begins to whisper in her ear in detail what you would do if you had both sex. If she can't take it anymore, go to her using the oral sex technique I mentioned above and then massage her deep spot with your middle finger. If you do it right, he will be very lucky after this happiness.

It's very important that you have great sex. It can create or disrupt relationships. If you break her in the bedroom, she has no reason to cheat or think about other boys.

Here are two things you need to do to make your girlfriend become sexual:

You have to stay long during sex. Premature ejaculation is the main cause of the girl's terrible sex. If you can't last long, you're in trouble.

But there are certainly solutions to this problem. They usually need to start working for a few weeks, but exercises that work with the ejaculatory muscle are excellent for a long time. When you have control of this muscle, you can live much longer and prevent premature ejaculation. If you continue the exercises, you can eventually continue as long as you want.

Remember, it is necessary to find out how your friend is sexually satisfying. Premature ejaculation is often the reason why women seek other sexual partners. It is extremely important to control ejaculation so they can experience the incredible orgasms they deserve.

This is the second most important factor for your girl to sleep:

You need to learn diversity. This means everything from different situations, from different predictive techniques to different sexual techniques such as oral sex.

There seems to be a lot, but it's not hard and you don't have to learn all at once. It's getting better. It is possible to learn how a new technique, or two a week, is a great fit for diversity for an incredible gender.

The same thing to do over and over is a sexual relationship that is very boring and boring. Again, this is sufficient reason for women to seek their sexual pleasures and fantasies elsewhere. Why would you get them to fantasize about something else and offer them the variety and sexual tension they can handle?

Prediction is a sexual structure and it is very important to build tension before sincerity comes. Now real business (real sex) is more than just a missionary position. There are many different and exciting sexual aspects that you can practice, such as changing speed and reaching your hands during a personal relationship. There is also oral sex that women love to find, but you need to take the time to learn how to do it the right way to create orgasms that augment the mind.

These changes and long-term factors are very important for sexual pleasure of love. Learn new and exciting tricks to motivate them and learn how to live as long as possible while having sex.

There are many people who have occasionally had sexual dysfunction. Long hours at work may require tax and reduce sexual desire for several days, which is best for us. A little relaxation and everything is back to normal. For some people, the problem is a little more serious.

Having a hypoactive sexual desire means that someone has little or no interest in sexual activity. Age, health and sexual interests will be considered before being classified as a sexual disorder.

Factors that indicate a noticeable sexual disorder are a high level of anxiety, relationship problems, or lack of attraction. Poor sexual techniques or discomfort can have a huge impact on libido. Everyone has different sexual needs, so one has to determine whether the lack of sexual interest is a disorder or is related to events in a person's life.

Another common problem is sexual arousal and orgasm disorder. In women, sexual arousal during contact is a problem and is defined as the inability to achieve orgasm after sex. There is a problem with erection in men. In short, no body is having fun!

Sexual attraction is important in any healthy relationship. It's no secret that a good sex life helps one relax and better cope with stress. Sex is a way to show your partner how you care for them. If your relationship has sexual disorders, seek the advice of a sexual therapist and don't bother. He or she may be able to give a jump back to his step and put a smile on his face.

Imagination can be a great way to increase sexual pleasure for you and your partner. Imagination can be used alone, with a partner or even in a group. With imagination you can go anywhere, be everyone and do everything. In some ways, the use of imagination is the best possible sexual technique. It's cheap, it's easy, it's yours and best of all, the world becomes yours and you're a champion.

Fantasies vary greatly from one person to another. Some fantasies relate to past lovers, friends or even people you've never met in person. Other fantasies are more related to the surroundings; in a lighthouse, under a bed, in a car, etc. Fantasies can target someone of the same sex, you and / or an inanimate object.

There are no rules. Sometimes people feel concerned about their fantasies because they do not include their partner. If so, you can best deal with your emotions by focusing on the positive effects these fantasies have on your sexual fantasy and your partner's relationships.

How does sexual fantasy of women differ from male?

Fantasies about men and women are actually more similar to each other than usual. Both sexes most often fantasize about confidentiality with their current partner. Men's fantasies are often more visual and come more quickly to sexual acts. Women include more foreplay and more palpable stimulation.

No big surprises, right? More importantly, female fantasies tend to focus on the dynamics of character relationships, while men are more often about impersonal sexual escapades. For example, both men and women may be physically enthusiastic about the hot graphics you see in porn movies, for example, but women don't tend to report being enthusiastic about explicit images unless their emotions are included.

The most common male fantasies are:

- Making love with an existing partner
- Giving and receiving oral sex
- Making love with more than one person
- Be dominant
- Be passive and submissive
- To experience the past experience
- See how others love each other
- Try new sexual positions

The most common female fantasies are:

- Making love with an existing partner
- Giving and receiving oral sex
- Making love with a new partner
- Romantic or exotic places
- Doing things not acceptable
- Be submissive
- To experience the past experience
- Found irresistible
- Try new sexual positions

Notifications when sharing fantasies

Although some couples feel that sharing and executing their fantasies has increased trust and intimacy, others don't.

Fantasies are very personal. Its disclosure is associated with certain risks, especially for someone you care for. Consider how you can do it if you don't like your imagination, or if you try to do it and it just doesn't work.

There is a powerful technique that will make your wife easier in orgasm. It will also ensure that your hair helps strengthen her orgasms. Although I am the first to say that you should not believe in the golden technique to satisfy a woman, I think this particular technique is the exception;

You can see why gold technology can attract the art of attention. Sexual sexual techniques would not normally work for all women. This is because most women have a choice when they want to encourage you.

But the art of care is not the same as other techniques in that it is not an exciting physical technique, but a technique that will help you choose the kind of physical simulation your wife needs.

By learning what your wife wants in the bedroom, you can use the right techniques to help her achieve her wishes and fantasies.

Regarding the art of paying attention to his master, focus on learning how to listen and watch your partner during a sexual session. It provides all the secrets you need to find out what she likes and dislikes.

Unfortunately, most men are too busy doing some type of technique and just watching and listening. Through the art of paying attention you will be able to learn so many powerful techniques. Not only that, but you will learn when a woman's special technique will be used to help her have strong orgasms.

Make a consistent orgasm for the woman and make sure the first three parts of this series are under your control. Otherwise, this last paragraph will not be as effective as it could be.

The biggest challenge I have noticed for the men I have trained is that they think they need all the techniques and work available in the sex world. They think they should persuade a woman of things that interest them.

And if they don't expect to know sexual techniques, they owe them the amount of their package.

When she was, she didn't care about the various aspects you know. And your package doesn't have as many decorative effects as you think. (Yes, it can help if you're well equipped. But remember what you need)

When it comes to big sex, the most important thing for a woman is your ability to move regularly from each other, maintain a good rhythm, watch continuous work and stay long enough. (All these things are under your control)

The first thing I want to discuss is your ability to stay long enough. Note that it doesn't say you can spend hours.

You don't have to wait an hour. If your work is done well, think about the first three parts of this series and if you're learning to build best practices ... you can create an orgasm for a woman in minutes.

A woman can suffer quickly. The correct pieces must be in place.One of the most important pieces in this area is your ability to predict creation using preliminary work. No need for verbal predictions ... need not be disturbed.

Good work falls under the category of "thinking *". (This is a technical term en route)

Something as simple as a very cold throat can cause limbs and can think of all the harmful things you can do. And the idea is so simple that it drains the juice and brings it to a very high level.

This may be an exaggerated example, but it will surprise you how many women can be excited at this level.

Sensual massage is usually the most versatile and effective form. It doesn't have to be long, but if you can set the squares in the right areas ... get rid of his orgasm.

The best areas to look for are neck, shoulders, lower back, buttocks and thighs. Based on my personal experience and hundreds of testimonials, these are the most common erogenic belts of a woman's body. The buttocks and thighs are particularly effective because they are so close to where the female body is ultimately.

The intention is to send a mental state that literally waits for sexual intercourse to begin. The more you can increase this expectation, the easier it is to create an orgasm.

And when you understand enough, try to find her favorite spot (what you learned if you did part 2 of this series) and maintain a good rhythm.

If you don't know how to dance, you can learn better.

I dance several times and a woman came to me and said something like, "If you can move your clothes like that, I don't think what you can do about it."

Women love a man who can dance. It's not because they want to dance constantly - whatever they have - but because a good dancer reminds a woman because it has a rhythm.

So if you don't know how to dance ... learn ... instantly.

I can confidently say that if you read and understand this book and the previous book in this series, you are in a much better position to give your wife an orgasm. (no pound suggested) And in terms of rhythm ...

If you don't know how to dance, you can learn better.

I dance several times and a woman came to me and said something like, "If you can move your clothes like that, I don't think what you can do about it."

Women love a man who can dance. It's not because they want to dance constantly - whatever they have - but because a good dancer reminds a woman ...

... because it has a rhythm.

So if you don't know how to dance ... learn ... instantly.

I can confidently say that if you read and understand this book and the previous book in this series, you are in a much better position to give your wife an orgasm.

# CONCLUSION

Biologically, sexual intercourse or intercourse refers to the penis of a man who enters the female vagina for reproductive purposes. Sexual intercourse is traditionally considered to be the natural end of any sexual intercourse between a man and a woman.

Today, however, this term is extended to include vaginal intercourse (with vaginal penis penetration causing ejaculation in men and female orgasm) and intercourse (with the oral strike of male or female genital organs). . It has also been extended to a wider range of behaviors and a wider range of motivation and intent - not just reproduction.

Pleasure in relationships for both sexes is one of the most intense behavior between two people, and for many it is one of the most intense physical stimuli that creates a comfortable and emotionally close relationship and closeness to others. Even the feeling that their partner has in women who fail to achieve orgasm during sexual intercourse.

The disadvantage, however, is that people, especially men, will do everything they consider "temporarypress Compared to sexual intercourse.

This puts great pressure on acquiring men and causes the woman to achieve orgasm through sexual intercourse. However, men and women can enjoy much more sexual intercourse if they accept pressure and consider it one of the many ways of making love. They should not consider all sexual activity as a nightmare, but in time to explore the great miracles of this friendly, terrible and wonderful experience to the point where they feel they have a very deep sexual connection that they feel are done.

Here are some good tips on how to improve intercourse, including ways to satisfy and satisfy intercourse.

**Pay attention to each other's body**

Avoid rushing to sex with immediate attention to the genitals. Conversely, take it easy, bow, pamper and learn to massage each other. Hang on to the body of another with gentle, kind and light snacks. Make sure your partner knows you find him attractive and desirable, creating a level of comfort and confidence. Kissing during sexual intercourse also increases connection and pleasure, which increases the likelihood of both reaching the peak. Use good foreplay with lots of lubrication.

## Add new techniques to your sexual intercourse

Any action, no matter how comfortable and satisfactory, can be repetitive tiring. The antidote is to add a good dose of expectation, excitement and surprise in ways that express your evolving sex style and unique personality in strengthening your sexual relationship.

## Avoid mechanical performance

Needless to say, the most important movement of sexual intercourse is always to push in and out. However, the formula used by most men in sexual intercourse often causes their partners to experience pain or discomfort rather than pleasure, and a general lack of interest in future sexual intercourse. The generality of men once in a woman simply begins with a quick and strong blow with regular blows. Instead, one should start slowly, very slowly, and build pace when switching deep moves with low moves.

## Different speeds and rhythmic forces

Slow down and then speed up. Then restart it. There is no change in the speed of pressure, and one places great emphasis on the experience and makes a variety of movements with hip rocking and cycling.

These movements can help a person discover the hot spots of his partner because the woman has different vaginal entry areas with special pressure sensitivity. The best working movements are pelvic cracks and slow circular movements. This is because the pelvic abdomen helps stimulate women's clit.

**Change your tasks**

Sexual gymnastics often interferes with you. Both sides should be the most important priority in sexual selection. The woman tries to control the show by going to the beginning - starting with a mission style - changing the dynamics of life. These feelings are different, love is spreading again.

However, ongoing changes in the overall situation of sexual tension can be reduced. Partners need to explore different situations and integrate them into their sexual activity by choosing people they think are more comfortable and work best.

**Practice Kegel exercises**

Pubococcygeal muscles (PC), which are both men and women, can function like any other muscle and, if toned, increase orgasm and sexual enjoyment. Tinted PC muscles that amplify naturally, enhance orgasmic intensity, better control over how soon a crop is extracted, and extend the time a person can create.

It's an easy way to recognize your computer's muscles and cone exercises when sending and releasing urine at startup.

A woman can do cone exercises to help her maintain her vaginal tone and function. For a woman, the exercise of the cone will strengthen her pelvic floor and restore the density she may have lost due to birth, age, or other factors. Generally, when a person strains the muscles of his computer, his penis jumps up and down. A good male workout is to place a washcloth on a stiff cock and raise your cock.

## Practice delay techniques

For women, the longer sex they last, the better they feel, as tensions may gradually increase. However, most men have occasional bad or slow erections and many of them suffer from premature ejaculation.

To help a person maintain and maintain an erection for better sexual intercourse, they practice delaying techniques such as squeezing (where a person, when he thinks ejaculate, he or his partner pushes just under his head); start-and-stop (where the man stops bumping as soon as ejaculation threatens and continues to reduce tension); and tightening (where it will stretch the muscles at the base of the penis as soon as there is a risk of ejaculation).

## Touch the clit during intercourse

For some women, the man's hand or mouth may be more intimate than sexual intercourse on their genitals. However, for most women, further stimulation during sexual intercourse is perfectly normal and stimulation of her clitoris during sexual intercourse is best.

A position that can stimulate a woman's clit when her partner pulls is good for her to have an orgasm. The position where she has control often gives her the most direct stimulation. A woman can be encouraged to masturbate during sexual intercourse, or her partner can do so using the techniques she uses.